Table of Contents

What could be a gluten-free slim down? 8

Who ought to eat a gluten-free eat less? 9

Can you go gluten-free to lose weight? 11

Are there dangers to attempting a gluten-free count calorie? 12

Will I go through gluten withdrawal in the event that 13

How do I get begun with a gluten-free slim down? 13

Delightful Gluten-Free Supper Formulas the Complete Fam 14

1. One-Pan Coconut-Lime Chicken 16

2. Classic Stuffed Peppers 18

3. Cacio E Pepe Sweet Potato Noodles 21

4. Lemony Chicken & Potatoes With Feta 23

5. Feta & Herb-Crusted Salmon 25

6. Rich Gochujang White Chicken Chili 28

7. Chili Cheese Sweet Potato Casserole 30

8. Moment Pot Pork Puttanesca 33

9. Best-Ever Gluten-Free Pasta 35

10. Corny Chorizo, Chickpea & Fresh Rice Skillet 38

11. Mushroom, Spinach & Gruyère Stuffed Pork Tenderloin ...41
12. Buckwheat Galettes with Ham & Egg 44
13. Wed Me Chicken 47
14. Crispy Chipotle Chicken Tacos 49
15. Tuscan Butter Shrimp 53
16. Fricasseed Halloumi Serving of mixed greens 55
17. Spinach Stuffed Chicken Breast 57
18. Cauliflower Pizza Outside 59
19. Discuss Fryer Pork Chops 61
20. Saag Paneer 63
21. Lobster Risotto 66
22. Chile Verde 69
23. Italian Sausage & Pepper Frittata Affogato 72
24. Garlicky Lemon Mahi-Mahi 74
25. Pastelón 76
26. Cauliflower Baked Ziti 81
27. Shrimp & Corn meal 84
28. Za'atar Sheet-Pan Chicken 87
29. Firecracker Salmon 90
30. Snap Tofu Grain Bowls 92

31. Vegetable Paella (Paella Verdure) 97
32. Slow-Cooker Rich Chicken & Potato Soup 99
33. Heated Pineapple Salmon 102
34. Caprese Chicken & Polenta Prepare 104
35. Reuben Bowls 106
36. One-Pan Chicken and Quinoa 109
37. Chicken Tostadas 112
38. Coconut Curry Salmon 114
39. Gazpacho with Burrata 117
40. Gazpacho with Burrata 119
41. Esquites Corn Chowder 121
42. Garlic Butter Meatballs & Zoodles 124
43. Chipotle-Lime Chilaquiles 126
44. Stuffed Pepper Casserole 128
45. Moment Pot Pho 131
46. Arepas 136
47. Ratatouille Casserole 138
48. Best-Ever Mexican Tostadas 140
49. Nectar Mustard Chicken 143
50. Heated Risotto with Lemon, Peas & Parmesan 147

51. Butternut Squash Curry 149

52. Coconut Curry Shrimp & Peas 151

53. Burrata Serving of mixed greens 154

54. Broiled Chickpea and Avocado Serving of mixed greens 156

55. Dark Bean Tostadas 159

57. Slow-Cooker Ruddy Wine Meat Stew 162

58. Zucchini Lasagna Roll-Ups 165

Budget-Friendly Gluten-Free Suppers 167

59. Herb-Grilled Chicken Frites 167

60. Skillet Buffalo Chicken 169

61. Ancient Bay Salmon with Lemony Squashed Peas 171

62. Dark Bean-Cauliflower "Rice" Bowl 173

63. Gluten-Free Teriyaki Chicken with Broccoli 175

64. Stuffed Heated Potatoes with Pesto & Eggs 177

Solid Soup Formulas 178

65. Slow-Cooker Spiced Lentil Soup with Vegetables 178

66. Tinola (Filipino Ginger-Garlic Chicken Soup) 180

67. Chunky Cheeseburger Soup 182

68. Classic Chicken Soup 184

69. Sweet Potato-Peanut Bisque 186

70.	Petit Fours	188
71.	Bunny Cake	194
72.	Parmesan-Crusted Cabbage Steaks Are the Most	198
73.	Gluten-Free Ice Cream Sandwiches	201
74.	Gluten-Free Apple Pie	203
75.	Gluten-Free Brownies	207
76.	Aperol Spritz Trifle	209

What could be a gluten-free slim down?

A gluten-free eat less excludes any foods that contain gluten, which may be a protein found in wheat and a few other grains. It suggests eating in a manner of speaking whole sustenances that don't contain gluten, like normal items, vegetables, meat and eggs, as well as taken care of without gluten sustenances like without gluten bread or pasta.

"Gluten may be a protein actually happening in certain nourishments, but it can too be added to nourishments amid handling for texture," clarifies Rajagopal. Gluten can be utilized as an official specialist and flavoring, so you'll in some cases discover it in nourishments you wouldn't anticipate. In expansion to nourishments like pizza, pasta, cereal and prepared merchandise, gluten can be in everything from soy sauce and ice cream to certain solutions, excellence items and dietary supplements.

A few individuals think going gluten-free implies not eating any carbohydrates, but this isn't the case. Parts of nourishments that contain carbs, such as rice, potatoes and beans, do not contain gluten.

Who ought to eat a gluten-free eat less?

Individuals with celiac illness

A gluten-free slim down is fundamental for individuals with celiac malady, an immune system reaction to gluten that causes the body to assault the small intestine, causing paunch torment, sickness, bloating or the runs. Individuals with celiac infection can't endure gluten in any form, and ought to take after a gluten-free diet for the rest of their lives. In case you have got celiac and inadvertently eat gluten, you'll likely experience the same indications you did some time recently you went gluten-free.

Individuals with gluten sensitivity

Another condition which will incite somebody to cut gluten from their diets may be a non-celiac gluten affectability, some of the time called gluten bigotry. "We don't have a clear definition for gluten narrow mindedness or a clear way to clarify it," says Rajagopal.

"We realize that a couple of people eat something that contains gluten and after that they don't feel great."

It's important not to accept that gastrointestinal disturbance is the result of gluten. In case you think you'll have a gluten bigotry, Rajagopal prescribes working with a doctor and a registered dietitian to urge to the foot of your side effects.

"There isn't a test for gluten bigotry, so we might attempt a prepare of disposal such as the moo FODMAP diet," says Rajagopal. This is often a transitory eating arrange that disposes of parts of nourishments that can bother the intestine, including wheat-based products. On the off chance that gluten is the source of the bothering, you will notice an advancement in symptoms such as:

- Bloating
- Stoppage or loose bowels
- Fatigue
- Gas
- Stomach torment

Individuals who are unfavorably susceptible to wheat

Individuals with a wheat sensitivity ought to dodge certain nourishments containing gluten, but not because of the gluten. Wheat triggers a safe reaction in their bodies, which can cause side effects such as a skin hasty, cerebral pain or wheezing. They can in any case eat gluten in different grains, including grain and rye.

Can you go gluten-free to lose weight?

Individuals who receive a gluten-free diet often lose weight, but it's ordinarily since they moreover cut out a part of handled nourishments and refined carbohydrates that contain gluten. In the event that you stop eating gluten to lose weight, it's critical to observe your parcel sizes, get normal exercise and eat bounty of entirety nourishments such as natural products, vegetables and incline proteins.

Are there dangers to attempting a gluten-free count calorie in case you do not have celiac illness?

If you cut all gluten out of your eating regimen, quite possibly's you just may pass up nutritious entire grains, fiber and micronutrients. Getting sufficient entirety grains in your diet is particularly vital if you're at chance for heart malady or diabetes. Entirety grains can lower cholesterol levels and indeed help regulate your blood sugar. In expansion, a few gluten-containing nourishments are sources of critical vitamins and minerals, such as B vitamins, press and magnesium.

Keep in intellect that some prepared gluten-free nourishments contain tall sums of undesirable ingredients such as sodium, sugar and fat. Expending these nourishments can lead to weight pick up, blood sugar swings, tall blood pressure and other issues. So, a gluten-free name doesn't essentially make a nourishment sound.

On the off chance that you don't have celiac malady or gastrointestinal disturbance, Rajagopal suggests evacuating profoundly prepared nourishments from you eat less some time recently expelling gluten. Include in more natural products, vegetables, whole-grain bread or pasta, and incline proteins. Numerous individuals discover they feel way better fair by eating way better, not by evacuating gluten.

Will I go through gluten withdrawal in the event that I begin eating gluten-free?

There's no logical prove to recommend that individuals really go through "withdrawal" when they halt eating gluten. Some individuals report feeling dizziness, nausea, extreme starvation and indeed uneasiness and depression when they all of a sudden go from eating a parcel of gluten to being gluten-free. These symptoms usually go absent after a few weeks on a gluten-free slim down, but conversation to your wellbeing care provider if they endure.

How do I get begun with a gluten-free slim down?

On the off chance that you're fascinated by trying a gluten-free diet, conversation to a doctor or an enlisted dietitian. Keep in acumen that some pre-arranged without gluten sustenance's They can direct you toward a changed eating orchestrate that meets your fascinating dietary requirements. contain tall amounts of bothersome fixings like sodium, sugar and fat.

Tips for making dietary changes in the event that you have got celiac infection incorporate:

Check for warnings on bundles. Numerous items that do not contain gluten may have been prepared in a office where there are gluten items.

Keep kitchen utensils, dishes and other nourishment prep things that are utilized for gluten-containing nourishments partitioned from your utensils.

Examined fixing names carefully to check for any follows of wheat. A few manufactured colors and seasonings moreover contain gluten.

Substitute oat, buckwheat, quinoa or other gluten-free or elective grain flours for wheat flour in cooking and baking.

Delightful Gluten-Free Supper Formulas the Complete Family Will Adore

Living gluten-free does not cruel you've got to skip out on your favorites. Distant from it! No shock, we're all around having our pasta, pizza, and tacos and eating them as well. So whether you're celiac, attempting to accommodate party guests, or basically requiring to cut out gluten, we've got bounty of astounding formulas that you will be astounded fair happen to be gluten-free (like our one-pan coconut lime chicken). The huge win? You'll still eat all the leading comfort nourishments like stuffed peppers, Instant Pot pho, and hand crafted gluten-free pasta without feeling like you're lost out on anything.

When it comes to making gluten-free formulas, you're progressing to need to be careful for a few fixings which will appear safe but really contain gluten. Soy sauce, which contains gluten, comes in a gluten-free adaptation, and you'll utilize tamari in a squeeze for all those stir-fries. Tortilla chips are about continuously gluten-free, much obliged to corn as a base. Worcestershire sauce, which you'll require for our Reuben bowls, is nearly continuously gluten-free, but do see out for malt vinegar (which does contain gluten).

Presently that you just know what to see out for, you'll be able get to cooking up our formulas for Moment Pot pork puttanesca, chili cheese sweet potato casserole, and feta & herb-crusted salmon. $5 says no one indeed takes note you made a totally gluten-free devour!

In case you ever pondered what exactly is gluten and what happens to your body after you go gluten-free, we've got tons of convenient guides about this strange protein. For more gluten-free thoughts, check out all our favorite gluten-free sweets, gluten-free appetizers, gluten-free breakfasts, and gluten-free sides.

1. One-Pan Coconut-Lime Chicken

In the event that our creamy Tuscan chicken could be a backbone at your house, this formula is aiming to be fair the thing to shake up your weeknight supper schedule. We combined quick-cooking chicken cutlets with a spicy-sweet coconut drain sauce that's out-of-this-world delicious. Tomatoes (and tomato glue) bring it back down to Soil, so you'll be able make this over and over (and over!) once more. Not persuaded? Did we say this comes together in fair one container, in less than thirty minutes?!

Fixings

- 6 chicken cutlets (almost 1 1/2 lb. add up to)
- 1 tsp. sweet paprika
- 1 tsp. kosher salt
- 1/4 tsp. naturally ground dark pepper
- 2 tbsp. coconut oil or vegetable oil
- 1 little yellow onion, finely chopped
- 1 little jalapeño, stemmed, seeded, finely chopped
- 3 cloves garlic, finely chopped
- 4 tsp. finely cleaved stripped ginger (from 1 [2"] piece))
- 2 huge, ready beefsteak tomatoes, seeded, finely chopped (around 2 c.)
- 1 tbsp. tomato paste
- 1 (15-oz.) can unsweetened coconut drain
- 1 tbsp. light brown sugar
- 1/4 c. fresh cilantro takes off, coarsely chopped
- 1 tbsp. new lime juice

Step 1

Season chicken done with paprika, salt, and pepper. In a huge, high-sided skillet over medium-high warm, warm 1 tablespoon oil. Working in batches, cook chicken, turning halfway through, until golden brown on both sides and close to cooked through, 1 to 2 minutes per side. Exchange to a plate.

Step 2

In same skillet over medium-high warm, warm remaining 1 tablespoon oil. Cook onion, mixing every so often, until somewhat delicate and fair turning brilliant, approximately 5 minutes. Include jalapeño, garlic, and ginger and cook, mixing, until fragrant and light brilliant, around 1 miniature more. Include tomatoes and tomato paste and cook, mixing sometimes, until tomato is softened and tomato glue is lightly toasted, approximately 2 minutes more.

Step 3

Include drain and brown sugar and bring to a bubble, blending until sugar is broken down. Settle chicken into skillet and return to a bubble. Bubble until chicken is cooked through, around 1 diminutive more.

Step 4

Remove from heat. Blend in cilantro and lime juice.

2. Classic Stuffed Peppers

Here at Delish, we're enormous fans of stuffed peppers (and it's no mystery as to why). Solid sufficient to hold their shape, peppers are large enough to hold a conventional sum of filling whereas taking to a assortment of flavors—they're the culminate vessel for countless combinations and ingredients. This versatile meal isn't only simple to make, but bolsters families huge and little, making it a cheap and simple weeknight dinner legend. Whereas we cherish to test with endless varieties, this classic recipe is difficult to defeat. Read on to find fair why this can be one of our fan-favorite recipes (one of our beat of 2022), at that point utilize it as a jumping-off point to make you possess dream stuffed peppers.

Ingredients

- 1/2 c. raw white or brown rice
- 2 tbsp. extra-virgin olive oil, furthermore more for sprinkling
- 1 medium yellow onion, chopped

- 3 cloves garlic, finely chopped
- 2 tbsp. tomato glue
- 1 lb. ground hamburger
- 1 (14.5-oz.) can diced tomatoes
- 1 1/2 tsp. dried oregano
- Legitimate salt
- Freshly ground dark pepper
- 6 chime peppers, tops and centers expelled
- 1 c. destroyed Monterey jack
- Chopped new parsley, for serving

Headings

Step 1

Preheat stove to 400°. In a small saucepan, get ready rice concurring to bundle informational.

Step 2

In the meantime, in a large skillet over medium heat, warm oil. Cook onion, stirring occasionally, until softened, almost 7 minutes. Stir in garlic and tomato glue and cook, mixing, until fragrant, around 1 minute more. Incorporate ground hamburger and cook, separating meat with a wooden spoon, until presently not pink, something like 6 minutes. Deplete abundance fat.

Step 3

Mix in rice and diced tomatoes; season with oregano, salt, and pepper. Let stew, mixing every so often, until liquid has reduced slightly, about 5 minutes.

Step 4

Arrange peppers cut side up in a 13"x9" preparing dish and sprinkle with oil. Spoon meat blend into each pepper. Beat with cheese, at that point cover preparing dish with thwart.

Step 5

Heat peppers until tender, about 35 minutes. Reveal and proceed to prepare until cheese is bubbly, approximately 10 minutes more.

Step 6

Top with parsley some time recently serving.

3. Cacio E Pepe Sweet Potato Noodles

Looking to change over a spiralizer veggie cynic Make them these cacio e pepe yam noodles Heaved in rich dim pepper sauce and showered with Parmesan and Pecorino, these yam noodles are flavorful to the point that nobody will for sure think practically asking for "customary" pasta.

Sweet potato noodles aren't troublesome to work with, but they're unquestionably not a coordinate one-for-one swap for wheat pasta. Here are some tips you'll need to be beyond any doubt as you travel toward sweet potato noodle nirvana.

Fixings

- 2 tbsp. extra-virgin olive oil, separated
- 12 oz. spiralizer sweet potatoes (sweet potato noodles), cut approximately 12" long
- 1 1/2 tsp. (or more) legitimate salt
- 1 tbsp. unsalted butter
- 1 tsp. crisply ground dark pepper, furthermore more
- 1/2 c. finely destroyed Parmesan (around 1 oz.), furthermore more for serving
- 1/2 c. finely destroyed Pecorino Romano (approximately 1 oz.)

Bearings

Step 1

Orchestrate all prepped and measured fixings inside simple reach of the stove. (The cooking in this formula goes rapidly, so it's basic to have everything prepared some time recently starting.)

Step 2

In a medium nonstick skillet over medium-high warm, warm 1 tablespoon oil. Include potato noodles and salt and cook, hurling every so often, until marginally mellowed but still a bit crunchy, 2 to 3 minutes.

Step 3

In the interim, in an expansive skillet over medium-low warm, liquefy butter with remaining 1 tablespoon oil. Include pepper and cook, whirling dish, until fragrant, 30 seconds to 1 minute.

Include noodles, Parmesan, and Pecorino and toss just until combined; season with salt, in the event that required.

Step 4

Separate noodle blend among bowls. Best with more Parmesan and pepper.

4. Lemony Chicken & Potatoes with Feta

Revive up an exemplary dish, lemon chicken and potatoes, by spooning the first delightful olive, almond, and parsley sauce over beat. Arranged from the dish drippings, the sauce is so basic to create without getting out an additional pot. The finest portion? This whole formula is made in fair one dish, making supper (and cleanup) simpler than ever. Essentially expel the chicken and potatoes to a serving platter once they're cooked, at that point mix the sauce fixings right into the container drippings. Liberally spoon the rich sauce over everything and serve!

Fixings

- 1 1/2 lb. child potatoes, split
- 1 lemon, closes trimmed, daintily cut, seeds evacuated
- 3 tbsp. extra-virgin olive oil, isolated
- Legitimate salt
- Naturally ground dark pepper
- 2 1/2 lb. bone-in, skin-on chicken thighs (almost 8)
- 1 tsp. sweet paprika
- 2 cloves garlic, finely chopped
- 1/2 c. chopped new parsley leaves
- 1/2 c. set Kalamata, Castelvetrano, or mixed olives, split
- 1/2 c. toasted cut almonds
- 1/4 c. white wine vinegar
- 4 oz. feta (almost 1 c.)

Bearings

Step 1

Preheat stove to 425°. In a 13"by-9" getting ready dish, fling potatoes, lemon, 2 tablespoons oil, 1/4 teaspoon salt, and many drudgeries of pepper. Broil until potatoes just start to turn brilliant, 14 to 16 minutes.

Step 2

Pat chicken dry with paper towels; season all over with 1 1/2 teaspoons salt and 1/4 teaspoon pepper. Settle chicken skin side up between potatoes. Sprinkle chicken with paprika and sprinkle with remaining 1 tablespoon oil.

Step 3

Broil chicken until skin is brilliant brown and an instant-read thermometer embedded into thickest portion (without touching bone) registers 165° and potatoes are fresh and brilliant brown, around 35 minutes.

Step 4

Utilizing tongs or an opened spoon, exchange

chicken and potatoes to a platter. Carefully mix garlic into hot skillet drippings (there ought to be around 1/2 glass drippings). Include parsley, olives, almonds, vinegar, and 1 teaspoon salt; blend to combine.

Step 5

Spoon sauce over chicken and potatoes. Crumble feta over best.

5. Feta & Herb-Crusted Salmon

We get it, salmon can be a little… threatening. Believe us, though you've fair gotta discover the cooking strategy that works for you. One of our favorites? Covering an entire angle, instead of individual filets, with fun toppings to include flavor all on fair one sheet container. For this Mediterranean-inspired adaptation, you just arrange your salmon on a sheet plate (lined with aluminum thwart for the least demanding cleanup), sprinkle on the garnishes, and prepare it for 25 minutes. No flipping, no staying, and no mess!

Fixings

- Cooking splash
- 1 expansive salmon filet (almost 2 1/4 lb.)
- 3/4 tsp. legitimate salt
- 1/4 tsp. crisply ground dark pepper
- 1/4 c. mayonnaise
- 1 1/2 c. disintegrated feta (around 7 oz.)
- 1/4 c. chopped new parsley
- 2 tbsp. chopped new dill
- 1 tsp. finely ground lemon get-up-and-go
- 1 clove garlic, finely chopped

- Lemon wedges, for serving

Headings

Step 1

Preheat broiler to 400°. Line a expansive heating sheet with thwart and oil with cooking spray.

Step 2

Orchestrate salmon substance side up on arranged sheet; season tissue side with salt and pepper. Spread mayonnaise over substance side.

Step 3

In a medium bowl, hurl feta, parsley, dill, lemon pizzazz, and garlic fair to combine, leaving feta in disintegrates. Sprinkle over mayonnaise.

Step 4

Bake salmon until fair cooked through and substance effortlessly pieces with a fork, almost 25 minutes. Serve warm with lemon wedges nearby.

6. Rich Gochujang White Chicken Chili

This rich, red-tinted turn on white chicken chili consolidates gochujang for a one of a kind turn on a classic winter supper. Gochujang, an umami-packed Korean ruddy chili glue that's both sweet and savory, gives parts of chili flavor without including a ton of heat, meaning this may be delighted in by everybody within the family (indeed the spice-averse).

Fixings

- 1 tbsp. extra-virgin olive oil
- 1 little yellow onion, finely chopped
- 3 cloves garlic, meagerly cut
- 2 tbsp. stripped finely cleaved ginger (from 1 [2"] piece)
- 4 c. low-sodium chicken broth

- 2 boneless, skinless chicken breasts (approximately 1 lb. add up to), cut into half crosswise
- 2 (15-oz.) cans cannellini beans, depleted and flushed
- 4 oz. cream cheese, cubed
- 1 (4.5-oz.) can green chiles
- 1/4 c. gochujang
- 1 tsp. dried oregano
- 1 tsp. ground cumin
- Kosher salt
- Crisply ground black pepper
- 1 (10-oz.) sack solidified corn (approximately 1 1/2 c.)
- 1/4 c. chopped fresh cilantro clears out, also more for serving
- 1 1/2 tsp. toasted sesame oil
- Tortilla chips, acrid cream, destroyed cheddar, kimchi, cut scallion, and sesame seeds, for serving

Headings

Step 1

In an expansive pot over medium warm, warm olive oil. Include onion and cook, blending once in a while, until softened, 8 to 10 minutes. Include garlic and ginger and cook, mixing, until fragrant and light brilliant, around 2 minutes.

Step 2

Pour in broth. Incorporate chicken, beans, cream cheddar, green chiles, gochujang, oregano, cumin, 1 1/4 teaspoons salt, and several drudgeries of pepper. Bring to a bubble, at that point decrease warm to medium and stew until chicken is delicate and fair cooked through, 10 to 12 minutes.

Step 3

Exchange chicken to a plate and shred with 2 forks. Crush almost one-quarter of beans in chili with the back of a spoon. Return destroyed chicken to pot and include corn. Bring to a stew and cook until chicken and corn are warmed through, 4 to 6 minutes. Expel from heat and blend in cilantro and sesame oil.

Step 4

Scoop chili into bowls Beat with tortilla chips, acrid cream, cheddar, kimchi, scallions, sesame seeds, and more cilantro.

7. Chili Cheese Sweet Potato Casserole

On the off chance that you think each bowl of chili ought to be covered up beneath hills of melty cheese and a big dollop of acrid cream, at that point this can be the casserole for you. With simmered sweet potatoes and dark bean chili layered together beneath a gooey cover of cheese, this simple vegan supper is both fantastically comforting and surprisingly healthy. Also, it's unendingly versatile just like numerous of our favorite casseroles, you'll truly play around with this recipe and make it you possess. Keep reading on for all our recommendations on making this weeknight savior:

Fixings

- 4 tbsp. vegetable oil, divided, additionally more for dish
- 3 medium sweet potatoes (around 1 1/2 lb. add up to), peeled and cut into 1/2" 3d shapes
- 1 1/2 tsp. legitimate salt
- 1 yellow onion, finely chopped
- 1 ruddy chime pepper, seeds and ribs evacuated, finely chopped
- 2 cloves garlic, finely chopped
- 1 tbsp. chili powder

- 1 tbsp. ground cumin
- 1 tsp. dried oregano
- 1 (14.5-oz.) can dark beans
- 1 (14.5-oz.) can diced tomatoes
- 1 (14.5-oz.) can tomato sauce
- 1 c. new or solidified corn parts
- 2 c. destroyed Colby Jack cheese
- 2 scallions, cut (approximately 1/4 glass)
- Acrid cream, for serving

Directions

Step 1

Preheat stove to 400°. Rub a 13"- by-9" glass baking dish with oil. On a heating sheet, hurl potatoes, 2 tablespoons oil, and 1/2 teaspoon salt.

Step 2

Cook potatoes until lightly browned and cooked through, 15 to 20 minutes. Let cool marginally. Diminish stove temperature to 350°.

Step 3

In the interim, in a huge skillet over medium warm, warm remaining 2 tablespoons oil. Include onion and 1/2 teaspoon salt and cook, blending once in a while, until somewhat mellowed, 3 to 4 minutes.

Include bell pepper, garlic, chili powder, cumin, and oregano and cook, blending once in a while, until pepper is fair marginally relaxed and flavors are fragrant, approximately 2 minutes more. Blend in beans, tomatoes, tomato sauce, corn, and remaining 1/2 teaspoon salt and cook, blending once in a while, until warmed through, 1 to 2 minutes.

Step 4

Pour half of chili into arranged dish. Sprinkle with half of potatoes. Best with remaining chili and potatoes.

Step 5

Cover with foil and heat casserole until bubbling around the edges and hot within the center, 20 to 25 minutes. Reveal, best with cheese, and proceed to heat until cheese is dissolved, 4 to 6 minutes more.

Step 6

Sprinkle with scallions and serve with acrid cream alongside.

8. Moment Pot Pork Puttanesca

It's lovely self-evident that we adore our Moment Pot for almost anything, but one region it truly exceeds expectations in is braised meat sauces like ragùs. Tougher cuts of meat (just like the pork bear here) that would take 2 1/2 hours on the stovetop or within the stove as it were take 30 minutes (!!!) within the Moment Pot and still come out super-tender.

Fixings

- 3 1/2 lb. skinless, boneless pork bear, abundance fat trimmed and disposed of, pork cut into 2" pieces
- Legitimate salt
- Crisply ground dark pepper
- 1 tbsp. extra-virgin olive oil
- 6 cloves garlic, peeled
- 2 oil-packed anchovy filets
- 1/4 c. tomato glue
- 1 (28-oz.) can entire peeled tomatoes
- 1/3 c. set Castelvetrano and/or Kalamata olives, divided
- 1/4 c. pressed new basil clears out, generally chopped, furthermore more for serving
- 2 tbsp. ruddy wine vinegar
- 1 tbsp. capers, depleted

- 1/2 tsp. smashed ruddy pepper pieces
- 1/2 tsp. granulated sugar
- Cooked polenta and shaved Parmesan, for serving

Headings

Step 1

Season pork with 1/2 teaspoon salt and 1/4 teaspoon dark pepper.

Step 2

In a Moment Pot, warm oil on Sauté 2 minutes. Include garlic and cook, blending as often as possible, until light brilliant, almost 2 minutes. Blend in anchovies and tomato paste and cook, blending, until tomato glue somewhat obscures and anchovies are broken up into small bits, around 2 minutes more.

Step 3

Include tomatoes and any juices, breaking up tomatoes with a wooden spoon. Include olives, basil, vinegar, capers, ruddy pepper chips, and sugar and mix to combine. Settle in pork.

Step 4

Near and bolt cover. Cook on tall weight 30 minutes, or until pork is exceptionally delicate.

Step 5

Physically discharge weight. Utilizing tongs, exchange pork to a expansive bowl. Utilizing 2 forks, shred pork Return pork to pot with sauce and set to Sauté. Bring to a stew and cook, blending once in a while, until sauce thickens, 8 to 10 minutes more.

Step 6

Serve pork over polenta. Beat with Parmesan and basil.

9. Best-Ever Gluten-Free Pasta

Yes, it's Genuine! You'll make astonishing without gluten pasta without any preparation, and it's not for sure troublesome! Underneath, check out our FAQs, at that point go forward and make the most prominent GF pasta of all time.

- 2 1/3 c. gluten-free flour, such as Cup4Cup
- 2 tsp. xanthan gum
- 1 tsp. legitimate salt
- 5 expansive eggs

Headings

Step 1

In a huge bowl, whisk together gluten-free flour, xanthan gum, and salt.

Step 2

Make a huge well within the center of your flour mixture and include eggs. Employing a fork, beat eggs until blended, at that point gradually coordinated flour into eggs until no dry flour is left and a ball of mixture has shaped. (You will have to be switch from a fork to your hands close the conclusion of the blending handle.)

Step 3

Turn batter out onto a gently floured surface and manipulate until smooth, 2 to 3 minutes.

Step 4

Cut mixture into quarters and wrap all but one in plastic wrap. On a gently floured surface, roll revealed mixture into a long rectangle almost 1/4" thick. Set pasta creator to most extensive setting and pass the rolled out mixture through 2 times. Overlay the brief closes of the batter to meet within the center of the rectangle, at that point crease in half so that the mixture is in quarters. Roll out once more to the batter is 1/4" thick, at that point pass through pasta creator 2 more times.

Step 5

Alter pasta maker to be 1 degree more limit and repeat handle. Proceed rolling, collapsing, and altering until craved thickness is come to. Batter should be somewhat translucent.

Step 6

Put rolled out dough onto a delicately floured surface and tidy with more flour. Rehash handle with remaining batter quarters.

Step 7

Alter pasta producer to desired width of noodles and nourish batter through machine. Partition noodles into similarly measured parcels and twist into homes. Put on a material lined heating sheet and cover with a clean kitchen towel until prepared to cook.

Step 8

To cook:

bring an expansive pot of salted water to a bubble and include pasta. Bubble, mixing delicately with a wooden spoon, until delicate, 2 to 3 minutes.

Step 9

Deplete and serve with your favorite pasta sauce.

10. **Corny Chorizo, Chickpea & Fresh Rice Skillet**

Crunchy and golden and on the off chance that you don't know it as of now, you'll after making this recipe crispy rice is a completely brilliant way to appreciate rice. Particularly when it turns into a crust and supports a truly delightful corny chorizo and chickpea filling. Crisping rice in a little olive oil includes an excellent textural contrast to steamed rice and extra flavor as the rice crisps and turns brilliant.

Fixings

- 1 1/3 c. water
- 1 c. jasmine rice
- Legitimate salt
- 3 tbsp. extra-virgin olive oil, partitioned
- 4 oz. dried Spanish-style chorizo, chopped into little pieces

- 1 small sweet onion, finely chopped (around 1 c.)
- 1 medium ruddy chime pepper, stemmed, seeded, and chopped
- 3 cloves garlic, daintily cut
- 1 (15-oz.) can chickpeas
- 3/4 c. dry white wine
- 1 (15-oz.) can diced tomatoes
- 1 1/2 tsp. sweet paprika
- 1 tsp. dried oregano
- 1/4 c. chopped new cilantro clears out, also more for serving
- 1 1/2 c. Mexican-style destroyed cheese (around 6 oz.)

Headings

Step 1

Combine water, rice, and 1/4 teaspoon salt in a little pan. Bring to a bubble over medium-high heat. Diminish heat to moo, cover, and stew until rice is delicate and fluid is ingested, 16 to 18 minutes. Expel from heat, uncover, and let sit at room temperature until prepared to utilize.

Step 2

Meanwhile, preheat broiler to 425°. In a medium (10") nonstick skillet over medium-high warm, warm 1 tablespoon oil. Include chorizo, onion, chime pepper, and garlic and cook, blending once in a while, until vegetables are tender, 6 to 8 minutes. Include chickpeas, wine, and 3/4 teaspoon salt. Bring to a bubble and cook, mixing sometimes, until wine is generally ingested, around 5 minutes.

Step 3

Include diced tomatoes and any juices, paprika, and oregano. Diminish warm to medium-low and stew, smashing around one-quarter of chickpea blend and tomatoes with the back of a spoon, until sauce is thickened, 4 to 6 minutes. Rub chorizo blend into an expansive heatproof bowl and blend in cilantro. Wipe skillet clean.

Step 4

In same skillet over medium-high warm, warm remaining 2 tablespoons oil until shining. Include rice to skillet. Utilizing the back of a measuring glass or spoon, press rice into foot and up sides of skillet, like a pie crust. Cook, undisturbed, until bottom of rice is brilliant and fresh, 4 to 6 minutes.

Step 5

Warm broiler. Fill center of rice hull with chorizo-chickpea mixture and sprinkle cheese over best. Broil until cheese is dissolved and brilliant, 1 to 2 minutes. Sprinkle with cilantro.

11. Mushroom, Spinach & Gruyère Stuffed Pork Tenderloin

Fast-cooking pork tenderloin could be a standard in our weeknight supper revolution, but that doesn't cruel we let it gotten to be so schedule that it gets to be boring. Instep, we mix it up every week with a combination of assorted flavors and courses of action, and this super stuffed mushroom, spinach, and Gruyère pork tenderloin absolutely does that.

Fixings

- 4 cuts bacon, chopped
- 8 oz. cremini mushrooms, daintily cut
- 1 little yellow onion, chopped
- 2 tbsp. extra-virgin olive oil, partitioned
- Legitimate salt
- Naturally ground dark pepper
- 2 cloves garlic, finely chopped

- 2 tsp. chopped new thyme takes off
- 2 c. pressed child spinach
- 1/4 c. dry white wine
- 1 1/2 c. destroyed Gruyère (almost 6 oz.)
- 1 pork tenderloin (approximately 1 1/2 lb.), trimmed
- Chopped new parsley, for serving

Headings

Step 1

In a medium skillet over medium warm, cook bacon, blending sometimes, until firm and fat is rendered, 6 to 8 minutes. Exchange bacon to a plate. Deplete all but 1 tablespoon fat from skillet.

Step 2

Return skillet to medium-high warm. Include mushrooms, onion, 1 tablespoon oil, 1/4 teaspoon salt, and 1/4 teaspoon pepper and cook, blending every so often, until vegetables are delicate, 6 to 8 minutes. Include garlic and thyme and cook, mixing, until fragrant, almost 1 diminutive. Pour in wine and cook, blending, until dissipated, around 1 miniature more. Include spinach and cook, hurling, until spinach is fair shriveled and any dampness is ingested, approximately 2 minutes. Evacuate skillet from warm and blend in Gruyère and bacon. Let cool somewhat.

Step 3

Preheat broiler to 425°. Butterfly pork by cutting the long way through the center without cutting through to the other side. Overlay open like a book and put between 2 sheets of plastic wrap. Employing a meat tenderizer, smooth to a meager 1/2" thick.

Step 4

Evacuate best piece of plastic wrap. Season pork on both sides with 3/4 teaspoon salt and 1/4 teaspoon pepper. Spread mushroom blend over cut side of tenderloin in an indeed layer. Beginning on long conclusion, firmly roll tenderloin to encase mushroom blend. Secure with kitchen twine and put on a heating sheet. Brush with remaining 1 tablespoon oil.

Step 5

Heat pork until an instant-read thermometer embedded into thickest portion registers 145°, 25 to 30 minutes. Let cool 10 minutes some time recently cutting.

Step 6

Exchange pork to a platter. Best with parsley.

12. Buckwheat Galettes with Ham & Egg

Like their sweet cousins, crêpes, galettes salute from Brittany, France. Since they're made with buckwheat flour, galettes are nuttier than crêpes, making them idealize for matching with savory fillings.

Here, they're loaded up with the exemplary ham, egg, and cheddar blend, known as "galette complete" in French. These buckwheat galettes with ham and egg are an extraordinary speedy supper or a centerpiece for breakfast or brunch. Match the galettes with a side serving of mixed greens dressed in a lively vinaigrette, and take after them up with something tres français like tarter tatin or chocolate mousse.

Fixings

- 3/4 c. entirety drain
- 1/4 c. all-purpose flour
- 1/4 c. buckwheat flour
- 8 expansive eggs, partitioned
- 4 tbsp. unsalted butter, 2 tbsp. dissolved, 2 tbsp. room temperature, separated
- Legitimate salt
- 8 oz. exceptionally meagerly cut Dark Forest-style ham
- 2 c. destroyed Gruyère (around 8 oz.)

- Crisply ground dark pepper
- Chopped new parsley or chives, for serving

Headings

Step 1

Preheat broiler to 375°. In a medium bowl, whisk drain, all-purpose flour, buckwheat flour, 2 eggs, 2 tablespoons liquefied butter, and 1/4 teaspoon salt.

Step 2

In a 10" nonstick skillet over medium warm, soften 1 teaspoon butter. Include a level 1/4 glass hitter and tilt skillet, twirling to convey hitter in an indeed, lean layer over foot of container. Cook until galette is set and light brilliant in places, approximately 1 miniature. Flip and proceed to cook until set and light brilliant on foot side, 30 seconds to 1 miniature more. Exchange to a plate. In case galette is cooking as well fast, reduce warm to medium-low. Rehash with remaining butter and player until you have got 6 galettes, stacking on plate as you go.

Step 3

Working with one at a time, put galette on a expansive rimmed preparing sheet. Beat with ham (almost 3 cuts, depending on how daintily it's cut), lining up with edge of galette or fair slightly overhanging. Sprinkle 1/3 glass cheese within the center of galette. Make a well in cheese. Split 1 egg into well; season with a squeeze of salt and pepper. Fold up 4 sides of galette over white portion of egg to form a square, taking off yolk and a few white uncovered. Rehash with remaining galettes, ham, cheese, and egg, orchestrating side by side on preparing sheet.

Step 4

Prepare until eggs are fair set and yolks are still runny, 13 to 15 minutes. Sprinkle with parsley and serve warm.

Step 5

Make Ahead:

Galette hitter can be made 12 hours ahead. Cover bowl and refrigerate.

13. Wed Me Chicken

Numerous of you've got likely listened of Ina Garten's "Engagement Cook Chicken" before, but this, in case I may say, is so much more delicious. When Delish editors begun eating up this dish, individuals begun shouting out marriage proposal-adjacent acclaims for this velvety, savory chicken supper ("I'd wed you for that chicken," and "Goodness MY GOD THAT'S MARRIAGE Fabric," were a few of the favorites). Consequently, the title and this dish were born:

a chicken supper so great, you fair might get a proposition by the final chomp.

Fixings

- 3 tbsp. extra-virgin olive oil, partitioned
- 4 (8-oz.) boneless, skinless chicken breasts
- Legitimate salt
- Freshly ground dark pepper
- 2 cloves garlic, finely chopped
- 1 tbsp. new thyme takes off
- 1 tsp. smashed ruddy pepper pieces
- 3/4 c. low-sodium chicken broth
- 1/2 c. chopped sun-dried tomatoes
- 1/2 c. overwhelming cream
- 1/4 c. finely ground Parmesan
- Torn new basil, for serving

Headings

Step 1

Preheat broiler to 375°. In a expansive ovenproof skillet over medium-high warm, warm 1 tablespoon oil. Liberally season chicken with salt and dark pepper and cook, turning midway through, until brilliant brown, almost 5 minutes per side. Exchange chicken to a plate.

Step 2

Return skillet to medium warm and warm remaining 2 tablespoons oil. Stir in garlic, thyme, and ruddy pepper pieces. Cook, blending, until fragrant, around 1 miniature. Blend in broth, tomatoes, cream, and Parmesan; season with salt. Bring to a stew, at that point return chicken and any gathered juices to skillet.

Step 3

Exchange skillet to broiler. Prepare until chicken is cooked through and juices run clear when chicken is penetrated with a cut, 10 to 12 minutes.

Step 4

Best with basil.

14. Crispy Chipotle Chicken Tacos

Additional fresh on the outside and tacky on the interior, these tacos are so much fun to form and eat. Putting cheese specifically in your skillet might sound off-base, but it works! Utilize a nonstick skillet and provide it time to begin crisping some time recently messing with it.

On the off chance that you go to overlay your tacos in half and the cheese doesn't appear to need to stay to the tortilla, provide it another miniature and try again. When off warm, the cheddar starts to harden and crisps up, giving the surface of a crunchy taco shell, yet at the same extra cliché. You will be making tacos every night of the week after these.

Fixings

AVOCADO Farm SAUCE

- 1 avocado
- 1 jalapeño, seeded and chopped
- 2 cloves garlic
- 1/2 c. stuffed new cilantro
- 1/4 c. buttermilk
- 1/4 c. acrid cream
- Juice of 1 lime
- Legitimate salt
- Naturally ground black pepper

TACOS

- 1 tbsp. extra-virgin olive oil
- 1 medium yellow onion, chopped

- 3 cloves garlic, minced
- 1 lb. ground chicken
- 1 chipotle Chile in adobo sauce, slashed, in addition to 2 tbsp.
- adobo sauce
- 1 tsp. chili powder
- 1 tsp. cumin
- Legitimate salt
- Crisply ground dark pepper
- 3 c. destroyed cheddar, isolated
- 8 little corn tortillas
- New cilantro clears out, for serving

Headings

AVOCADO Farm SAUCE

Step 1

In a nourishment processor or blender, puree avocado, jalapeño, garlic, cilantro, buttermilk, acrid cream, and lime juice until smooth; season with salt and pepper.

Step 2

Exchange sauce to a waterproof holder. Refrigerate until prepared to utilize.

Step 3

Make Ahead:

Sauce can be made 3 days ahead. Keep refrigerated.

TACOS

Step 1

In an expansive skillet over medium heat, heat oil. Include onion and cook, blending, until mollified, almost 5 minutes. Include garlic and cook, mixing, until fragrant, almost 1 diminutive more. Include chicken and cook, breaking up meat with a wooden spoon, until now not pink, almost 8 minutes. Include chipotle Chile, adobo sauce, chili powder, and cumin; season with salt and pepper. Evacuate from warm.

Step 2

In a little nonstick skillet over medium warm, orchestrate about 1/4 cup cheese in a circle in an indeed layer almost the size of your tortillas. Put a tortilla on best. Spoon a few chicken filling on one half of tortilla and approximately 2 tablespoons cheese on the other half. Cook until cheese on foot begins to fresh, almost 4 minutes. Employing an elastic spatula, overlay the half with cheese up and over chicken, squeezing to assist taco stay closed. Cook until warmed through, almost 1 miniature, at that point flip and proceed to cook until other side is warmed through, almost 1 diminutive more. Exchange to a plate. Repeat with remaining tacos.

Step 3

Best tacos with cilantro. Serve with avocado farm sauce alongside.

15. Tuscan Butter Shrimp

What can't Tuscan butter progress? This velvety, flavor-packed sauce is the star of numerous of our weeknight supper favorites, from our Tuscan chicken (one of our most adored formulas) to our Tuscan butter gnocchi. When we're searching for switch up our protein or longing for a summer-worthy dinner we turn to this shrimp adaptation. The most excellent portion? Matched with sweet cherry tomatoes and spinach, this saucy shrimp dinner is prepared to be served in less than 30 minutes. Here's beginning and end you might want to be aware:

Fixings

- 2 tbsp. extra-virgin olive oil
- 1 lb. shrimp, peeled, deveined, and tails evacuated

- Legitimate salt
- Crisply ground dark pepper
- 3 tbsp. butter
- 3 cloves garlic, minced
- 1 1/2 c. divided cherry tomatoes
- 3 c. child spinach
- 1/2 c. overwhelming cream
- 1/4 c. naturally ground Parmesan
- 1/4 c. basil, meagerly cut
- Lemon wedges, for serving (discretionary)

Bearings

Step 1

In a colossal skillet over medium-high warm, warm oil. Season shrimp done with salt and pepper. When oil is sparkling but not smoking, include shrimp and burn until underside is brilliant, almost 2 minutes, at that point flip until murky. Expel from skillet and set aside.

Step 2

Diminish warm to medium and include butter. When butter has softened, mix in garlic and cook until fragrant, about 1 miniature. Include cherry tomatoes and season with salt and pepper. Cook until tomatoes are beginning to burst at that point include spinach and cook until spinach is starting to wilt.

Step 3

Blend in overwhelming cream, Parmesan and basil and bring mixture to a stew. Decrease warm to moo and stew until sauce is marginally diminished, almost 3 minutes.

Step 4

Return shrimp to skillet and blend to combine. Cook until shrimp is warmed through, embellish with more basil and press lemon on best some time recently serving.

16. Fricasseed Halloumi Serving of mixed greens

We think it's due time that halloumi, the brined Cypriot cheese, got its time within the highlight. Other than the delightfully squeaky surface (where the cheese curd significant others at?) and the tart, salty flavor, the tall softening point is truly what makes this cheese stand out; eaten crude it's as it was Alright, but when warm is connected, it creates a scrumptious brilliant hull.

Fixings

FOR THE DRESSING

- 2 tbsp. lemon juice
- 1/4 c. extra-virgin olive oil
- 2 tbsp. crisply chopped dill
- 2 tbsp. crisply chopped mint
- Legitimate salt
- Crisply ground dark pepper

FOR THE SALAD

- 1 c. canned chickpeas, washed and depleted
- 1 little head fennel, cored and thinly cut
- 1/4 c. green olives, such as Castelvetranos, set and generally chopped
- 2 tbsp. extra-virgin olive oil
- 8 oz. halloumi, cut into 1/4" slices
- 1 pita, torn into bite-sized pieces
- 2 c. freely stuffed arugula
- 1 medium maritime orange, cut into sections

- 1/2 ready avocado
- Ruddy pepper pieces

Bearings

Step 1

In an expansive bowl, whisk together all dressing fixings and season to taste with salt and pepper.

Step 2

Include chickpeas, fennel, and olives to bowl with dressing and hurl to combine.

Step 3

In an expansive skillet over medium warm, warm 1 tablespoon oil. Include halloumi and cook until charred and brilliant on both sides, around 4 to 6 minutes add up to. Expel cheese to a expansive plate.

Step 4

Within the same skillet over medium warm, warm remaining oil. Include pita and toast until brilliant and fresh, around 4 minutes. Evacuate to plate with halloumi.

Step 5

Include arugula, halloumi, and pita to bowl with chickpeas, fennel, and olives and hurl to combine. Remove peel and pit from avocado half on the off chance that vital and cut crosswise into lean cuts.

Step 6

Include orange portions and avocado cuts and hurl very gently until combined. Season to taste with salt, pepper, and ruddy pepper pieces, and serve.

17. Spinach Stuffed Chicken Breast

Our fantasy for this chicken came from us appreciate everything spinach artichoke and how well our primavera stuffed chicken comes out each time we make it. Hassel back your chicken by cutting shallow openings into your chicken breasts (do not cut all the way through!) and stuff each opening with bacon and a velvety spinach and artichoke filling. It'll make your weeknight chicken dinner sing! It's untraditional, but all the finest suppers are.

Fixings

- 4 boneless skinless chicken breasts
- Legitimate salt
- Naturally ground dark pepper

- 4 oz. cream cheese, softened
- 1/2 c. solidified spinach, defrosted, depleted, and crushed
- 1/3 c. chopped canned artichoke hearts
- 1 c. destroyed mozzarella, partitioned
- Squeeze smashed ruddy pepper drops
- 4 strips bacon, cut into 4 strips
- 2 tbsp. extra-virgin olive oil

Headings

Step 1

Preheat stove to 400°. Line an expansive heating sheet with foil. Make openings widthwise in chicken, being cautious not to cut all the way through chicken. Season with salt and pepper. Put on arranged heating sheet.

Step 2

In a medium bowl, combine cream cheese, spinach, artichokes, and ½ container of mozzarella. Season with salt, pepper, and a squeeze of ruddy pepper pieces. Fill each other opening with cream cheese blend and fill remaining openings with a chunk of bacon. Sprinkle remaining ½ cup mozzarella on best and sprinkle with oil.

Step 3

Heat until chicken is cooked through and bacon is crispy, 35 minutes.

18. Cauliflower Pizza Outside

Cauliflower has attacked kitchens all over. As a solid, clear slate it has taken the frame of pounded potatoes, toasty bread and indeed the center of our Thanksgiving table. Conceivably our favorite utilize of cauliflower as a culinary ace of mask is in pizza hull. It might sound insane but it can be a delicious and solid elective to the classic. In this simple, gluten-free pizza formula, you're essentially making cauliflower rice as base the base for your outside.

Fixings

- 1 expansive head cauliflower, generally chopped
- 1 expansive egg
- 2 c. destroyed mozzarella, divided
- 1/2 c. naturally ground Parmesan, partitioned
- legitimate salt
- 1/4 c. marinara or pizza sauce
- 2 cloves garlic, minced

- 1 c. grape or cherry tomatoes, divided
- Torn new basil, for serving
- Balsamic coat, for sprinkling

Headings

Step 1

Preheat oven to 425°. In a huge skillet, bring around 1/4" water to a boil. Season with salt. Remember cauliflower for one even layer and cook until fresh delicate, 3 to 4 minutes. Trade to a perfect kitchen towel (or paper towels) and press to exhaust water.

Step 2

Include depleted cauliflower to nourishment processor and beat until ground. Deplete overabundance water in paper towels.

Step 3

Exchange depleted cauliflower to an expansive bowl and include egg, 1 container mozzarella and 1/4 glass Parmesan, at that point season with salt.

Step 4

Exchange batter to a baking sheet lined with cooking shower and pat into a hull. Prepare until brilliant and dried out, 20 minutes.

Step 5

Beat outside with marinara, remaining mozzarella and Pram, garlic and tomatoes and heat until cheese is dissolved and crust is crisp, 10 minutes more.

Step 6

Decorate with basil and sprinkle with balsamic coat.

19. Discuss Fryer Pork Chops

In the event that you more often than not control clear of pork chops, at that point this formula is here to alter your mind it's a cheap and simple supper must. We understand we've had our reasonable share of overdone, dry pork chops. But, when cooked right, they can be succulent and ultra-flavorful, whereas still getting a slight fresh on the outside. That's where the enchantment of the discuss fryer co mess in. With our blend of seasonings and this helpful kitchen contraption, you'll be able have a for all intents and purposes hands-off supper in 20 minutes. Keep perusing on for all of our beat tips about how to form them the finest they can be:

Ingredients

- 4 boneless pork chops, around 1"-thick
- 2 tbsp. extra-virgin olive oil
- 1/2 c. finely ground Parmesan
- 1 tsp. garlic powder
- 1 tsp. legitimate salt
- 1 tsp. onion powder
- 1 tsp. smoked paprika
- 1/2 tsp. freshly ground dark pepper

Headings

Step 1

Pat pork chops dry with paper towels, at that point coat both sides with oil.

Step 2

In a medium bowl, combine Parmesan, garlic powder, salt, onion powder, paprika, and dark pepper. Coat both sides of pork chops with Parmesan mixture, squeezing to follow.

Step 3

In an air-fryer container, organize pork cleaves in a solitary layer. Cook at 375°, flipping midway through, until an instant-read thermometer embedded into thickest part of pork chop registers 145°, almost 9 minutes.

Step 4

Let pork chops rest around 10 minutes some time recently serving.

20. Saag Paneer

This vigorous curry is a staple in numerous Indian eateries. With a sensible fixing list, our own is easy to reproduce at home. Blocks of paneer are promptly available in numerous huge general stores.

Fixings

- 4 tbsp. canola or vegetable oil
- 8 oz. paneer or extra-firm tofu, cut into 1" blocks

- 1 little ruddy onion, generally chopped
- 6 cuts new ginger
- 4 garlic cloves
- 1 green serrano chile, seeds and white "vein" expelled in case you favor less heat
- 1 c. canned tomato sauce
- 1 tbsp. ground coriander
- 1 tsp. ground cumin
- 1/2 tsp. cayenne (¼ tsp. for less warm)
- 1/4 tsp. ground turmeric
- 1 tsp. legitimate salt
- 1 lb. infant spinach, finely chopped
- 1/2 c. water
- 1/2 c. overwhelming cream
- 1/2 tsp. gram masala
- Steamed white rice or naan (store-bought or hand crafted), for serving

Bearings

Step 1

In a huge nonstick or cast-iron skillet, heat 2 tablespoons oil over medium warm until it shines. Include the paneer in one layer and cook until brown on one side, almost 2 minutes. Flip and cook until brown on the opposite side, an additional 2 minutes. (The paneer will splatter, so use caution!) Transfer the paneer to a bowl filled with hot tap water to assist keep it delicate.

Step 2

Beat the onion, ginger, garlic, and Chile in a nourishment processor until minced. (You will have got to include a bit of water to the processor.)

Step 3

In a large Dutch broiler or pot, warm the remaining oil over medium warm until it shines. Include the onion glue and cook until light brown and a few of it sticks to the foot of the skillet, around 2 minutes.

Step 4

Mix within the tomato sauce, coriander, cumin, cayenne, turmeric, and salt. Lower the warm and stew, in part secured, for almost 8 minutes.

Step 5

Include spinach and cook, secured, until wilted, around 4 minutes. Blend in the water and simmer, secured, until spinach turns a pale green color, almost 15 minutes.

Step 6

Drain the paneer and include it to the spinach, in conjunction with the cream and gram masala. Proceed to stew the curry, secured, blending every so often, around 5 minutes.

Step 7

Serve warm nearby cooked rice or naan.

21. Lobster Risotto

Once you think of decedent suppers, there are few that can eclipse the rich, velvety, seafood-stuffed eminence that's lobster risotto. A basic combination of new aromatics, white wine, and fish stock changes humble Italian rice grains into the fantastic, tacky, tasty rice porridge that we've all come to adore. And including new, faintly sweet lobster meat is all that's required to require your risotto over the best.

Fixings

- 6 c. store-bought or custom made fish or lobster stock
- 4 tbsp. unsalted butter, partitioned
- 6 oz. cherry tomatoes, divided
- Legitimate salt
- 1 huge shallot, finely chopped
- 2 cloves garlic, cut
- 1 1/2 c. Arborio, vial one Nano, or carnaroli rice
- 1 c. dry white wine
- 2 oz. ground Parmesan, additionally more for serving
- 1/4 c. mascarpone
- 6 oz. cooked lobster meat, chopped
- 2 tbsp. finely chopped chives, also more for serving
- 1 tsp. finely ground lemon pizzazz
- Squeeze of pulverized ruddy pepper drops (discretionary)

Bearings

Step 1

In a little pot over medium low-heat, warm stock and cover pot to keep warm.

Step 2

In the meantime, in a huge, high-sided skillet over medium-high warm, dissolve 2 tablespoons butter. Include tomatoes and 1/2 teaspoon salt and cook, blending sometimes, until tomatoes begin to break down. Include shallot, garlic, and 1/4 teaspoon salt and cook, mixing every so often, until fragrant, almost 2 minutes more.

Step 3

Include 1 tablespoon butter and blend until dissolved. Include rice and decrease warm to medium. Toast rice in butter, blending once in a while, until rice starts to stay to foot of container and make high-pitched sizzling clamors, 2 to 3 minutes. Include wine and cook, mixing always, until fluid is vanished, almost 2 minutes.

Step 4

Scoop 4 ounces' warm broth into rice and blend continually until fluid is totally retained, almost 2 minutes. Proceed to include broth 4 ounces at a time, blending briefly, at that point permitting fluid to be completely retained after each expansion. After around 30 minutes, rice ought to be completely cooked with around 4 ounces' broth remaining. Evacuate pot from warm and blend in Parmesan, mascarpone, 1 teaspoon salt, remaining broth, and remaining 1 tablespoon butter. Crease in lobster meat, chives, lemon get-up-and-go, and ruddy pepper pieces, in the event that utilizing.

Step 5

Spoon risotto into bowls. Beat with chives and Parmesan.

22.   Chile Verde

Chile Verde may be a conventional dish from Northern Mexico that can be made with a few sorts of meat. Pork is classic, and here, you'll change a pork bear into meltingly delicate chunks through a long braise. This formula makes a big batch, idealize for serving at a supper party or a Cinco de Mayo celebration. No matter the event, Chile Verde sets well with margaritas and Mexican rice.

Fixings

- 2 lb. tomatillos (approximately 16), shucked and washed
- 3 huge poblano peppers, split the long way, stems and seeds expelled
- 3 cubanelle peppers, divided the long way, stems and seeds evacuated
- 1 to 2 serrano peppers, depending on your warm inclination

- 1 expansive white onion, cut into huge chunks
- 4 cloves garlic
- 3 lb. pork bear, cut into 1" pieces
- 2 tbsp. extra-virgin olive oil
- Legitimate salt
- 1 tsp. naturally ground dark pepper, additionally more to taste
- 2 tsp. ground cumin
- 2 tsp. dried Mexican oregano
- 1/2 tsp. ground coriander
- 3 c. low-sodium chicken broth
- Cilantro clears out, for serving
- Lime wedges, for serving

Bearings

Step 1

Preheat broiler to tall. On a huge rimmed preparing sheet, organize tomatillos, poblanos, cubanelles, serranos, onion, and garlic cloves in an indeed layer. Broil until vegetables are profoundly charred, flipping tomatillos and peppers midway, 10 to 15 minutes. (Observe closely.) Evacuate sheet from broiler and let vegetables cool.

Step 2

In the interim, warm a expansive Dutch stove over medium high. In a expansive bowl, season pork with the oil, 2 tablespoons salt, and 1 teaspoon pepper. Include pork to Dutch broiler in an indeed layer, and cook, undisturbed, for 5 minutes, or until one side is browned. Blend pork and smooth to an indeed layer, and cook undisturbed once more, around 5 minutes more. Proceed to cook, blending presently so pork gets browned all over, almost 5 minutes more.

Step 3

Include cumin, oregano, and coriander and blend so meat is equitably coated in flavors. Cook for around 30 seconds, or until the flavors are fragrant.

Step 4

In a blender, join seared vegetables, stock, and 1 tablespoon salt. Mix until smooth; pour into pot. Return the pork to the pot and increment warm to tall. When fluid fair starts to boil, reduce heat to moo.

Step 5

Cook, secured, mixing every so often, for almost 1½ hours, or until the pork falls separated effectively and the sauce has diminished and thickened.

Step 6

Evacuate cover, and cook revealed for an extra 45 minutes, blending frequently, until sauce has thickened encourage Season to taste with salt and pepper.

23. Italian Sausage & Pepper Frittata Affogato

Breakfast meets dinner in this marinara-and mozzarella-beat Italian hotdog and pepper frittata affogato. Fittingly, the Italian word "affogato" implies suffocated, which clarifies the marinara topping. It loans this dish a vibe some place between a breakfast frittata and pizza, meaning it's agreeable for beautiful much any feast of the day.

Take after it up with an affogato the Italian treat featuring gelato doused in espresso.

Fixings

- 12 expansive eggs
- 1/4 c. chopped new basil clears out, additionally more for serving
- 1/4 c. entire drain

- 1/2 tsp. legitimate salt
- 1/4 tsp. naturally ground dark pepper
- 2 tbsp. extra-virgin olive oil
- 1 medium ruddy chime pepper, stemmed, seeded, and thinly cut
- 1 little yellow onion, meagerly cut
- 1/2 lb. fiery or sweet Italian sausage, casings evacuated
- 2 c. store-bought or hand crafted marinara sauce
- 1 1/2 c. destroyed mozzarella (around 6 oz.)

Bearings

Step 1

Preheat broiler to tall. In a medium bowl, whisk eggs, basil, drain, salt, and pepper.

Step 2

In a 10" ovenproof nonstick skillet over medium-high, heat oil. Include chime pepper and onion and cook, mixing every so often, until fair delicate, approximately 3 minutes. Thrust vegetables to one side of skillet and include wiener to the other side. Employing a wooden spoon, break up wiener into little bits, at that point blend to combine with vegetables and cook, blending once in a while, until wiener is brilliant brown and cooked through and vegetables are delicate, 4 to 6 minutes.

Step 3

Pour egg blend into skillet with wiener and vegetables. Cook, gradually blending with a spatula and scratching foot and sides of skillet to make huge curds, until eggs are nearly set, 2 to 3 minutes. Spread into an indeed layer.

Step 4

Exchange skillet to stove and broil until brilliant in spots and puffed, almost 3 minutes. Expel from broiler. Spread marinara over and sprinkle with mozzarella. Continue to broil until sauce is warm and cheese is liquefied and bubbly, 3 to 5 minutes more. Let cool almost 5 minutes some time recently serving. Sprinkle with basil.

24. Garlicky Lemon Mahi-Mahi

Magnificently flaky and fragile when cooked, mahi is the fish supper you should make the entire year. The firm and mellow angle is not only totally scrumptious, but super-versatile you can heat, burn, barbecue, or broil it and best it with any number of distinctive sauces or dressings. Our favorite way to prep it? Cook it on the stove with a few new veg like asparagus, at that point cover it in a lemony butter sauce. Here's how to form it the leading it can be:

Fixings

- 3 tbsp. unsalted butter, separated
- 2 tbsp. extra-virgin olive oil, partitioned
- 4 (4-oz.) mahi mahi fillets
- Legitimate salt
- Crisply ground dark pepper
- 1 lb. asparagus, trimmed
- 3 cloves garlic, finely chopped
- 1/4 tsp. pulverized ruddy pepper chips
- 2 lemons, 1 cut, 1 zested and juiced
- 1 tbsp. chopped new parsley, furthermore more for serving

Headings

Step 1

In an expansive skillet over medium warm, warm 1 tablespoon butter and 1 tablespoon oil until butter is liquefied. Include mahi mahi; season with salt and dark pepper. Cook, turning sometimes, until brilliant on both sides, 4 to 5 minutes per side. Transfer to a plate.

Step 2

In same skillet over medium-high warm, heat remaining 1 tablespoon oil. Include asparagus and cook, hurling every so often, until delicate,

2 to 4 minutes; season with salt and dark pepper. Exchange to plate with angle.

Step 3

In same skillet over medium warm, liquefy remaining 2 tablespoons butter. Include garlic and ruddy pepper drops and cook, stirring occasionally, until fragrant, about 1 miniature, at that point mix in lemon cuts, pizzazz, and juice, and parsley. Evacuate from warm. Return mahi and asparagus to skillet and spoon sauce over.

Step 4

Beat with parsley some time recently serving.

25. Pastelón

Associated to a Puerto Rican lasagna, pastelón layers up firm fricasseed sweet plantains with melty mozzarella cheese and picadillo, a blend of ground hamburger, tomatoes, sofrito (more on that underneath), spices, briny olives, and a pop of pleasantness from raisins. It takes a bit to get ready all the components, but it's worth it for this sweet and savory dish you'll be able effectively serve to a swarm. (May we recommend going with a basic side?)

Fixings

FOR THE PLANTAINS:

- 2 c. canola oil
- 6 exceptionally ready plantains (almost 9 oz. each)
- Legitimate salt

FOR THE SOFRITO:

- 1 c. chopped yellow onion (almost 7 oz.)
- 1 c. chopped green chime pepper (almost 6 oz.)
- 1 1/2 c. new cilantro clears out and lean stems, generally chopped
- 6 cloves garlic

FOR THE PICADILLO:

- 2 tbsp. canola oil
- 1 1/2 lb. incline ground meat (85%)
- Legitimate salt
- 1/2 tsp. crisply ground dark pepper
- 2 tsp. sweet paprika
- 2 tsp. dried oregano
- 1 tsp. ground cumin
- 3 tbsp. tomato glue

- 1 (28-oz.) can diced, fire-roasted tomatoes
- 1 c. water
- 2 tbsp. yellow raisins
- 1/2 c. pimento-stuffed manzanilla olives, daintily cut

FOR THE TOPPING:

- 3 huge eggs
- 2 tbsp. entire drain
- 4 1/2 c. destroyed mozzarella

Headings

MAKE THE PLANTAINS:

Step 1

In an expansive pot over medium-high warm, warm 2 mugs oil (around 1-inch) until a profound broil thermometer peruses 350°. Sear plantains, working in clumps (approximately 4 per clump), until brilliant and delicate, flipping midway through, around 3 minutes. Utilizing tongs or a kitchen insect, exchange plantains to a paper towel-lined heating sheet and season with salt. Rehash with remaining plantains.

MAKE THE SOFRITO:

Step 1

In a nourishment processor, beat the onion, chime pepper, cilantro, and garlic until finely chopped.

MAKE THE PICADILLO:

Step 1

In a huge, high-sided skillet, warm the remaining 2 tablespoons of oil over medium-high warm. Rub the sofrito into the skillet and cook, mixing regularly, until the blend dries out and starts to turn brilliant, around 5 minutes.

Step 2

Include the meat to the skillet with the sofrito and season with 2 teaspoons salt, ½ teaspoon pepper, paprika, oregano, and cumin. Cook, employing a wooden spoon to break up the meat into little pieces, at that point mixing every so often until hamburger is evenly cooked and now not pink, about 7 minutes. Include the tomato glue and cook, blending, until toasted, around 2 minutes.

Step 3

Include the tomatoes, 1 container of water, and raisins to the skillet and bring to a bubble Decrease warm to medium and stew until thickened, something like 5 minutes. Evacuate from the warm and blend within the olives.

MAKE THE TOPPING:

Step 1

Whisk the eggs with the drain and season with ¼ teaspoon salt. Set aside.

Gather THE PASTELÓN:

Step 1

Preheat the stove to 350°. Arrange one-third of the plantains in an indeed layer (do not cover) within the foot of an 8"x"12 heating dish. Beat with half of the picadillo and 1 ½ mugs of the cheese. Rehash 1 time with another third of the plantains, the remaining picadillo, and another 1 ½ mugs of the cheese.

Step 2

Orchestrate the remaining third of plantains over pastelón and sprinkle the egg blend equally over best. Sprinkle remaining 1 ½ glass cheese over best, then bake until bubbly and cheese is brilliant, around 40 minutes. Let cool 15 minutes some time recently serving.

26.   Cauliflower Baked Ziti

Alright, fine. There's not really any ziti in this recipe. But you truly won't indeed take note. The broiled cauliflower does a strong work of supplanting the pasta. (P.S. It's moreover incredible at supplanting macaroni in our Stacked Cauliflower Prepare as well as our Keto Mac and Cheese.)

In a past version of this formula, we called for whitened cauliflower, which brought about in a looser, soupier sauce in the wake of examining client reviews and retesting, we've since redesigned the trimmings to call for seared cauliflower, which delivers a more regular ziti sauce consistency. Our favorite way to broil cauliflower? In an expansive bowl, hurl cauliflower with 2 tablespoons oil and season with salt. Spread cauliflower onto two huge heating sheets and cook at 375° until delicate and softly brilliant, 40 to 45 minutes.

Fixings

- 1 tbsp. extra-virgin olive oil
- 1 medium onion, chopped

- 2 cloves garlic, minced
- Squeeze pulverized ruddy pepper chips
- 1 lb. ground meat
- Legitimate salt
- Crisply ground dark pepper
- 2 tbsp. tomato glue
- 1 tsp. dried oregano
- 1 (28-oz.) can pulverized tomatoes
- 2 tbsp. meagerly cut fresh basil, additionally more for decorate
- 2 medium heads cauliflower, cut into florets, simmered
- 1 1/2 c. ricotta
- 2 c. destroyed mozzarella
- 1/2 c. crisply ground Parmesan

Bearings

Step 1

Preheat stove to 375°. In a huge, deep-sided skillet over medium warm, heat oil. Include onion and cook, blending once in a while, until delicate, 5 minutes. Include garlic and ruddy pepper drops and cook for 1 miniature. Include ground meat and season with salt and pepper. Cook until not pink, approximately 6 minutes. Deplete fat.

Step 2

Return skillet over medium warm and include tomato glue and oregano. Cook until stick hardly darkens, roughly 2 minutes more. Include tomatoes and bring to a stew. Diminish warm and cook, mixing until marginally decreased and flavors have melded, 10 to 15 minutes. Expel from warm and blend in basil.

Step 3

Put cauliflower in an expansive bowl and pour sauce on best. Blend until completely coated. Exchange half the cauliflower blend to a large heating dish and spread into an indeed layer. Dab all over with half the ricotta and sprinkle with half the mozzarella and Parmesan. Best with an indeed layer of the remaining cauliflower mixture and remaining cheeses.

Step 4

Prepare until cheeses are dissolved and brilliant, 25 to 30 minutes.

Step 5

Embellish with basil some time recently serving.

27. **Shrimp & Corn meal**

Wealthy and tacky, shrimp and corn meal is the comfort food staple we'll welcome all year long. On the off chance that you've never made corn meal some time recently, it can be troublesome to urge them fair right. Fortunately, we've tried this recipe once more and again to create beyond any doubt it's sheer flawlessness. Our formula is extra-creamy due to a liberal sum of cheese (in our book, no corn meal is total without) and butter. We too took this formula to the next-level by including in fresh bacon. Not as it were does this amp up the surface of our dish, but cooking our shrimp in bacon fat includes piles of flavor. The result may be a wealthy and wanton weeknight supper (or filling brunch!) we'll joyfully burrow into any time of year. Keep reading on for all of our best recommendations on how to culminate each step of this Southern staple:

Fixings

- 2 c. low-sodium chicken broth
- Legitimate salt
- 1 c. corn corn meal
- 4 oz. yellow cheddar, destroyed (approximately 1 c.)
- 4 tbsp. unsalted butter, cubed
- Naturally ground dark pepper

- 10 oz. thick-cut bacon, cut into 1/2" cuts
- 1 lb. expansive tail-on shrimp, peeled, deveined
- 2 cloves garlic, finely chopped
- 1 tsp. dried oregano
- 1/4 tsp. paprika
- 1 tbsp. tomato glue
- 3/4 c. vegetable broth
- 4 scallions, thinly sliced, also more for serving
- Juice of 1/2 lemon

Bearings

Step 1

In a medium pot, bring broth and 2 glasses water to a bubble; liberally season with salt. Diminish warm to medium-low and bring to a stew. Whisk in corn meal and cook, whisking always, until corn meal have ingested fluid and are exceptionally delicate, approximately 15 minutes. Mix in cheese and butter until melted; season with salt and pepper.

Step 2

In the interim, in an expansive skillet over medium warm, cook bacon, mixing sometimes, until fresh, about 8 minutes. Transfer bacon to a cutting board. Pour off everything except 2 tablespoons bacon fat. Chop bacon into little pieces.

Step 3

In a huge bowl, hurl shrimp with garlic, oregano, and paprika; season with salt. In same skillet over medium warm, cook shrimp, turning once in a while, until pink and cooked through, 4 to 6 minutes. Exchange shrimp to a plate.

Step 4

In same skillet over medium warm, cook tomato glue, stirring, until glue obscures, 1 to 2 minutes. Whisk in broth and bring to a stew. Cook, mixing occasionally, until sauce thickens and is diminished by almost half, 4 to 5 minutes; season with salt. Return shrimp to skillet and hurl to combine. Blend in scallions and lemon juice.

Step 5

Partition corn meal among plates. Beat corn meal with shrimp, sauce, bacon, and more scallions.

28.   Za'atar Sheet-Pan Chicken

Once you do not feel like doing a parcel of dishes, sheet-pan meals are your best companion. Whether you're longing for pork chops, gnocchi, or even chicken fajitas, a sheet dish guarantees to streamline your feast and take off you with negligible cleanup:

idealize for weeknights, a sluggish weekend meal—or any day at all.

We've made a part of awesome sheet-pan suppers, but this za'atar chicken formula is a modern favorite. Bone-in chicken thighs, infant potatoes, broccoli, and red onion are all hurled in a basic olive oil, lemon juice, and za'atar marinade, at that point simmered to firm, schmaltzy flawlessness. And fair to kick it up another score, we're sprinkling it all in a rich tahini sauce to wrap up it off.

Ingredients

- 3 tbsp. za'atar flavor mix
- 10 tbsp. extra-virgin olive oil, partitioned
- 6 tbsp. new lemon juice, separated
- 1 tbsp. furthermore 1 tsp. legitimate salt, isolated
- 4 skin-on, bone-in chicken thighs (approximately 2 lb. add up to)
- 1 lb. fingerling potatoes, split longwise
- 8 oz. broccoli, managed and cut into 1" florets
- 1 ruddy onion, cut into 1"-thick wedges

- 1/4 c. tahini
- 3 tbsp. cold water
- Lemon wedges, for serving

Bearings

Step 1

In an expansive bowl, whisk za'atar, 6 tablespoons oil, 4 tablespoons lemon juice, and 1 tablespoon salt. Exchange 1/4 glass marinade to a little bowl and set aside. Include chicken to remaining marinade and hurl to coat. Cover and let sit at room temperature 30 minutes.

Step 2

Preheat stove to 425°. Include potatoes to bowl with chicken and hurl to coat, at that point organize chicken skin side up and potatoes cut sides down on an expansive heating sheet. Pour any remaining marinade over. Prepare chicken and potatoes 15 minutes.

Step 3

In the meantime, in a medium bowl, hurl broccoli and onion with saved marinade, 2 tablespoons oil, and 1/2 teaspoon salt. Evacuate sheet skillet from stove. Transfer broccoli and onion to skillet, making beyond any doubt vegetables make contact with container as much as possible.

Step 4

Proceed to prepare until vegetables are delicate and chicken is cooked through (an instant-read thermometer embedded into thickest portion ought to enlist 165°), approximately 20 minutes more.

Step 5

In the interim, in a little bowl, whisk tahini, water, and remaining 2 tablespoons oil, 2 tablespoons lemon juice, and 1/2 teaspoon salt. Sprinkle over chicken and vegetables. Serve with lemon wedges alongside.

29.   Firecracker Salmon

If you're attempting to track down one more method for welcoming on the warm at dinnertime, this firework salmon recipe is here to brush the rooftop off your mouth. Affirm, not truly. The sweet and fiery firework sauce joins three super hot components sriracha, Chile drops, and new ginger for a layered way to deal with warm. Served here with salmon, the firecracker sauce would too be scrumptious on flame broiled shrimp, heated tofu, or prepared chicken breasts.

Fixings

- Cooking shower
- 1 (2-lb.) skin-on salmon filet
- 1/2 tsp. legitimate salt
- 1/4 tsp. crisply ground dark pepper
- 1/4 c. dim brown sugar
- 3 cloves garlic, minced
- 3 tbsp. sriracha
- 2 tbsp. extra-virgin olive oil
- 2 tbsp. new lime juice
- 1 tbsp. reduced-sodium soy sauce or tamari
- 2 tsp. sweet paprika
- 1 tsp. finely chopped peeled ginger
- 1/2 tsp. smashed ruddy pepper drops
- 1 scallion, chopped
- Lime cuts, for serving

Bearings

Step 1

Preheat stove to 350°. Line an expansive rimmed preparing sheet with thwart and oil with cooking shower.

Step 2

Orchestrate salmon skin side down on arranged sheet. Season flesh side with salt and dark pepper.

Step 3

In a medium bowl, whisk brown sugar, garlic, sriracha, oil, lime juice, soy sauce, paprika, ginger, and ruddy pepper chips. Coat tissue side of salmon with brown sugar blend.

Step 4

Prepare until salmon is cooked through, 20 to 24 minutes. Rub any sauce on sheet skillet over salmon, at that point best with scallions and lime cuts.

30. Snap Tofu Grain Bowls

There are few things as fulfilling as a grain bowl. Building a scaled down devour with a blend of proteins, garnishes, and sauces has gotten to be one of our favorite ways to eat (see Chipotle and all of the comparative build-a-bowl eateries). This veggie lover formula may be a bit of a culinary street trip through a few Jamaican staples:

sweet browned plantains, fragrant rice and peas, and tofu in a snap marinade. To include a touch of crunch, causticity, and color we beat it all off with a simple ruddy cabbage and carrot slaw that's just as tasty on its claim because it is within the bowls.

Fixings

FOR THE Fricasseed PLANTAINS

- 2 huge ripe plantains, slice on a bias into ½" pieces
- Vegetable oil for searing
- Legitimate salt

FOR THE CABBAGE CARROT SLAW

- 1 little ruddy cabbage, destroyed
- 1 expansive carrot, meagerly cut into matchsticks
- 1 tsp. legitimate salt
- 2 tbsp. extra-virgin olive oil
- 2 tbsp. apple cider vinegar
- Juice of 1 lime
- 1/2 tbsp. nectar
- 1/2 tbsp. Dijon mustard
- Legitimate Salt

- Crisply ground dark pepper

FOR THE Fast RICE & PEAS

- 1 (15-ounce) can ruddy kidney beans, undrained
- 1 (7-ounce) can coconut drain
- 2 scallions, split
- 10 allspice berries
- 3 cloves garlic
- 1/2 scotch cap pepper, seeds evacuated
- 2 sprigs thyme
- 1 c. basmati rice
- Legitimate Salt

FOR THE TOFU & BOWLS

1 medium onion, generally chopped

3 scallions, generally chopped also more cut for embellish

- 2-inch piece ginger, generally chopped
- 2 scotch cap peppers
- 3 sprigs thyme, clears out evacuated and stems discard
- 3 tsp. allspice, crisply ground in case possible, divided

- 1/4 c. low-sodium soy sauce
- 1/4 c. apple cider vinegar
- Legitimate salt
- Crisply ground dark pepper
- 1/4 tsp. cinnamon
- 1 tsp. garlic powder
- 2 (16-ounce) bundles additional firm tofu, depleted and squeezed
- Additional virgin olive oil
- Cilantro, finely chopped for decorate
- Lime wedges

Bearings

FOR THE Browned PLANTAINS

Step 1

Fill an expansive skillet with sufficient oil to fair cover the foot of the skillet with oil. Warm over medium-high until oil sparkles. Working carefully, include plantain cuts to dish in a single layer.

Step 2

Sear, turning half way through midway through, for 6 to 8 minutes. When the plantains are a profound brilliant brown and can be effectively punctured with a fork, evacuate to a paper towel lined plate and season with salt.

FOR THE CARROT CABBAGE SLAW

Step 1

In a huge bowl combine cabbage, carrots and salt and set aside for 15 minutes. Press the cabbage blend over sink to evacuate the dampness.

Step 2

In the meantime, in a little bowl, whisk olive oil, vinegar, lemon juice, nectar and mustard until completely combined. Season with salt and pepper to taste. Hurl cabbage with dressing to coat and chill.

FOR THE Fast RICE & PEAS

Step 1

In a medium pot over medium warm, include kidney beans, coconut drain and 1 container additionally 2 tablespoons water. Include scallions, allspice, garlic, scotch cap, thyme, a liberal squeeze of salt and dark pepper. Bring to a bubble at that point diminish to a stew and let cook revealed for 20 minutes.

Step 2

In a fine work strainer, flush basmati beneath cold water until the water runs clear. Expel the allspice, scallions and garlic. In the event that a parcel of fluid has vanished, refill to the initial level with water, at that point bring to a bubble. Include rice, diminish to a stew and cook covered for 15 to 20 minutes or until the rice is cooked through.

FOR THE TOFU AND BOWLS

Step 1

In a nourishment processor or blender, include onion, scallion, ginger, scotch cap, thyme, 2 teaspoons allspice, soy sauce and vinegar. Mix until a smooth paste has shaped. Season with salt and pepper and set aside in an expansive bowl.

Step 2

Cut tofu into ¼ cuts and sprinkle both sides with 1 teaspoon allspice, cinnamon, garlic powder, salt and pepper. Include tofu to the twitch marinade and carefully hurl to coat, making beyond any doubt to not break the cuts. Cover with saran wrap and chill for 2 hours and up to expedite.

Step 3

Preheat stove to 400°F and organize a rack within the best and center of your stove. On a material lined preparing plate, lay the tofu out in a single layer, making beyond any doubt a few of the marinade has followed to the cuts. Cook tofu on the center rack for 30 minutes until the tofu has browned on the edges and the snap flavoring has obscured somewhat. Move plate to the best rack and broil on tall for 2 to 3 minutes, or until the tofu has started to char in places.

Step 4

To serve, layer rice, 3 to 4 cuts of tofu, plantains and slaw in a huge bowl. Embellish with meagerly cut scallion, a sprinkle of cilantro, and lime wedges.

31. Vegetable Paella (Paella Verdure)

This veggie-pressed paella meets up in less than 60 minutes, and, without a doubt prevalent, the vast majority of the cooking occurs inside the oven. Briefly returning the skillet to the stovetop after heating is the key to achieving a firm rice hull on the foot, regularly alluded to as socarrat (meaning "burnt" in Catalan).

Fixings

- 4 tbsp. extra-virgin olive oil, isolated
- 2 medium zucchini, divided the long way and cut into half moons

- 8 oz. sliced mushrooms
- Legitimate salt
- 1/2 little yellow onion, finely chopped
- 3 cloves garlic, finely chopped
- 1 tsp. smoked paprika
- Squeeze saffron strings (discretionary)
- 1 (14-ounce) can chopped tomatoes
- 1 1/2 c short-grain paella rice, (for example, Bomba rice)
- 1 c. new or solidified peas
- 1 c. piquillo peppers, cut (or broiled ruddy peppers)
- 5 oz. child spinach
- 3 1/2 c. vegetable broth
- Chopped fresh parsley, for serving
- Lemon wedges, for serving

Bearings

Step 1

Preheat broiler to 425°F.

Step 2

In a profound 12-inch cast-iron or other ovenproof skillet, warm 2 tablespoons oil over medium warm. Include zucchini and mushrooms and season with salt.

Cook, undisturbed, until brilliant on one side, around 3 minutes. Hurl and cook, sitrring every so often, until brilliant and delicate, 8 to 10 minutes; transfer to a small bowl.

Step 3

To same skillet, include 2 tablespoons olive oil and return to medium warm. Include onion and season with salt. Cook, mixing regularly, until mellowed, 3 to 5 minutes. Include garlic, smoked paprika, and saffron and cook, stirring, until fragrant, 30 seconds. Include tomatoes and rice and blend to combine. Mix in zucchini blend, peas, piquillo peppers, and spinach, mixing to shrink spinach. Include broth and ¾ teaspoon salt. Bring to a bubble at that point carefully exchange to the broiler. Prepare, revealed, until fluid is ingested and rice is delicate, 20 to 22 minutes.

Step 4

Exchange skillet to stovetop over medium warm. Cook until foot of rice is fresh, 2 to 3 minutes. Let rest 5 minutes. Beat with parsley and serve with lemon wedges.

32. Slow-Cooker Rich Chicken & Potato Soup

A warm and velvety soup with exceptionally negligible exertion is our perfect supper. Prep everything within the morning and after that come domestic at night to this delightful soup that will please everyone. No require to burn or utilize any other skillet. It's healthy and filling and fair the thing you wish to life up your spirits. The moderate cooker makes the chicken absolutely drop isolated while making the potatoes rich and sensitive. Utilize your favorite curry powder to flavor up the dish and make it indeed more comforting. On the off chance that you aren't a fan of kale, you'll continuously utilize spinach or Swiss chard instep!

Fixings

- 1 1/2 lb. boneless, skinless chicken breasts
- Legitimate salt
- Crisply ground dark pepper
- 1 lb. infant yellow potatoes, quartered
- 1 (8-oz.) square cream cheese, relaxed
- 1 medium yellow onion, chopped

- 1 expansive carrot, chopped
- 1 jalapeño, finely chopped
- 4 cloves garlic, finely chopped
- 1 small bunch thyme
- 4 c. low-sodium chicken broth
- 1 c. entirety drain
- 1 tbsp. chicken bouillon glue
- 2 tsp. curry powder
- 1 tsp. dried oregano
- 1 bunch Tuscan kale, center ribs and stems evacuated, chopped (about 4 c.)

Headings

Step 1

Season chicken all over with salt and pepper and place in a moderate cooker. Include potatoes, cream cheese, onion, carrot, jalapeño, garlic, and thyme and mix to combine. Add broth, drain, bouillon, curry powder, and oregano; season with salt and pepper.

Step 2

Cover and cook on moo until chicken is delicate and falling separated, 5 to 6 hours. Exchange chicken to a plate and shred with 2 forks.

Return chicken to slow cooker and add kale. Blend until well combined.

Step 3

Proceed to cook on moo until kale is shriveled, almost 10 minutes more; season with salt and pepper, on the off chance that required.

33. Heated Pineapple Salmon

Giving the salmon a speedy broil at the conclusion of cooking gives the marinade a chance to caramelize it's as well great Fair make for certain to watch out for it, so you don't overcook the salmon! two to three minutes is all you would like beneath a hot broiler.

Fixings

- Cooking shower, for skillet
- 17 pineapple rings, new or canned

- 1 huge salmon filet (almost 3 lbs.)
- Legitimate salt
- Naturally ground dark pepper
- 3 tbsp. liquefied butter
- 3 tbsp. sweet chili sauce
- 2 tbsp. crisply chopped cilantro
- 3 cloves garlic, minced
- 2 tsp. crisply ground ginger
- 2 tsp. toasted sesame oil
- 1/2 tsp. smashed ruddy pepper pieces
- Toasted sesame seeds, for embellish
- Daintily cut green onions, for embellish
- Lime wedges, for serving

Headings

Step 1

Preheat stove to 350°. Line a huge rimmed preparing sheet with foil and oil with cooking shower. Within the center of the thwart, lay pineapple cuts in an indeed layer.

Step 2

Season both sides of the salmon with salt and pepper and put on best of pineapple cuts.

Step 3

In a little bowl, whisk together butter, chili sauce, cilantro, garlic, ginger, sesame oil, and ruddy pepper chips. Brush all over salmon filet.

Step 4

Heat until the salmon is cooked through, around 25 minutes. Switch the broiler to broil, and broil for 2 minutes, or until angle is somewhat brilliant. Embellish with sesame seeds and green onions and serve with lime wedges.

34. Caprese Chicken & Polenta Prepare

Gnocchi significant others, this dish is for you, but it encompasses a small spin rather than utilizing gnocchi made from potatoes, it's prepared with polenta gnocchi. Yes, polenta gnocchi could be a thing, and it's similarly as comforting and cravable. Additionally, our form is as simple because it gets, thanks to a basic need store easy route. We utilize store-bought polenta sold in tubes and cut it into rounds instead of making the gnocchi from scratch.

Fixings

- 4 lean chicken cutlets (almost 1 lb. add up to)
- 1/2 tsp. Italian flavoring
- Legitimate salt
- 1/4 c. extra-virgin olive oil, isolated
- 1 (18-oz.) tube pre-cooked polenta, cut into 1/2"-thick rounds
- 3 cloves garlic, minced
- 5 oz. child spinach (almost 5 pressed c.)
- 2 c. store-bought or custom made marinara
- 1/3 c. water
- 8 oz. bocconcini (little new mozzarella balls), daintily cut
- 1/2 c. pressed new basil clears out, thinly sliced

Headings

Step 1

Warm broiler to tall. Season chicken with Italian flavoring and 1/2 teaspoon salt.

Step 2

In an expansive straight-sided skillet over medium-high warm, warm 2 tablespoons oil. Organize polenta rounds in a single layer and cook until brilliant on the foot, approximately 2 minutes. Employing a lean metal spatula, flip polenta and continue to cook until brilliant on the other side, almost 2 minutes more. Exchange polenta to a plate.

Step 3

Decrease warm to medium (skillet will be hot from burning polenta) and warm 1 tablespoon oil. Add chicken and cook, flipping midway through, until brilliant brown on both sides and fair cooked through, about 2 minutes per side. Exchange to plate with polenta.

Step 4

Warm remaining 1 tablespoon oil over medium warm. Include garlic and cook, blending regularly, until fragrant, almost 10 seconds. Include spinach and cook, hurling, until fair shriveled, almost 1 miniature more. Pour marinara and water into skillet and blend to combine.

Step 5

Expel skillet from warm and tuck chicken and polenta into sauce. Best with bocconcini.

Step 6

Broil until cheese is dissolved, almost 3 minutes. Let cool 10 minutes. Beat with basil.

35. Reuben Bowls

The Reuben will continuously hold an extraordinary put in our hearts when it comes to our favorite classic sandwiches, but we'll be the primary to confess:

it's got a Part going on. Corned hamburger, Russian dressing, sauerkraut, and Swiss cheese are all unstably stuffed between two pieces of rye bread, and in the event that it's not impeccably wrapped from the store, you're in for a chaotic time. Skip all of that by making our Reuben bowls instep (same idea, easier execution). They've got all the flavors you cherish, in a helpful bowl culminate for any meal.

Fixings

FOR THE DRESSING

- 1/4 c. mayonnaise
- 2 tbsp. sweet pickle savor

- 4 tsp. ketchup
- 1 1/2 tsp. arranged horseradish
- 1 tsp. new lemon juice
- 1/2 tsp. Worcestershire sauce
- Legitimate salt
- Naturally ground dark pepper

FOR THE BOWL

- 2 tsp. caraway seeds
- 1 tbsp. extra-virgin olive oil
- 1/2 yellow onion, chopped
- 1/4 green cabbage, daintily cut (almost 5 c.)
- 1 c. destroyed carrot
- 3/4 lb. corned hamburger, cut 1/2" thick
- 1 1/2 c. sauerkraut, depleted
- 1 c. destroyed Swiss
- 1/4 c. meagerly cut cornichon
- 1 green onion, meagerly cut

Bearings

Step 1

Make the dressing:

In a little bowl, whisk together mayonnaise, pickle relish, ketchup, horseradish, lemon juice, and Worcestershire. Season with salt and pepper.

Step 2

Make the bowl:

In a huge skillet over medium-high warm, toast caraway seeds, blending, until fragrant, approximately 30 seconds. Exchange to a plate.

Step 3

Return skillet to medium-high warm and heat oil. Include onion and cook blending until delicately brilliant, approximately 3 minutes. Include the cabbage and carrot and season with salt and pepper. Cook, blending once in a while, until cabbage is crisp-tender, 5 minutes.

Step 4

Blend in corned meat and sauerkraut, hurling until warmed all through, 1 miniature more. Beat cabbage blend with Swiss cheese, cover, and cook until cheese is melty and bubbly, 3 minutes. Expel from warm.

Step 5

Scramble simmered caraway seeds and cornichon on best, then drizzle with dressing and decorate with green onion some time recently serving.

36.   One-Pan Chicken and Quinoa

Here's a speedy and simple supper that's tall in protein and takes exceptionally small exertion. We cherish the Tex-Mex flavors here; the chili powder and cayenne include a pleasant kick that the avocado and acrid cream superbly offset. Of course, feel free to use a small less of either flavor in the event that you favor.

Ingredients

- 2 lb. (almost 6) boneless, skinless chicken thighs
- 1 tsp. chili powder
- Kosher salt
- Crisply ground dark pepper
- 1 tbsp. extra-virgin olive oil
- 1 little yellow onion, chopped
- 1 poblano pepper, seeded and chopped
- 3 cloves garlic, minced

- 1 tbsp. tomato glue
- 1 c. low-sodium chicken broth
- 1 (14-oz.) can fire-roasted diced tomatoes
- 1 (14-oz.) can dark beans, depleted and washed
- 1 c. solidified corn, defrosted
- 1 c. dry quinoa
- 1 tsp. cumin
- 1 tsp. dried oregano
- 1/4 tsp. cayenne pepper
- Juice of 1 lime
- 1/4 c. naturally chopped cilantro
- 1 avocado, cut, for serving
- Acrid cream, for serving
- Lime wedges, for serving

Headings

Step 1

Season chicken thighs all over with chili powder, salt, and pepper.

Step 2

In an expansive skillet over medium-high warm, warm oil. Include chicken and cook until brilliant, around 4 minutes per side. Remove chicken from skillet and place on a plate.

Step 3

Decrease warm to medium and include onion and poblano pepper. Cook until soft, around 5 minutes, at that point include garlic and cook until fragrant, 1 miniature more. Include tomato paste and blend to coat veggies.

Step 4

Pour in broth and rub up any bits from the bottom of dish. Include tomatoes, beans, corn, and quinoa. Mix in cumin, oregano, and cayenne and season with salt and pepper. Return thighs to skillet. Bring blend to a bubble, at that point diminish warm and cook, secured, 20 minutes. Evacuate cover and proceed cooking, revealed, until quinoa is delicate and chicken is cooked through, 10 to 15 minutes more.

Step 5

Evacuate chicken from skillet, at that point blend in cilantro and lime juice.

Step 6

Serve quinoa with chicken, avocado, acrid cream, and lime wedges.

37. Chicken Tostadas

Here at Delish, we accept that tostadas fair can be the idealize weeknight supper. They have all the scrumptious crunch of a tortilla chip, but act as a sturdy vehicle for whatever toppings you like. Here, meaning rich hand crafted refried beans and chile-spiked destroyed chicken topping. We stack these up with plenty of toppings, but not so many that our tostadas can't carry them to our craved goal. Ready to form the most excellent chicken tostadas ever? Keep reading on for all of our beat tips:

Fixings

- 5 tbsp. neutral oil, isolated
- 1 expansive white onion, one-half finely chopped, one-half meagerly cut
- 1 tsp. ground cumin
- 3 tsp. legitimate salt, isolated
- 1 tsp. naturally ground dark pepper, partitioned
- 2 (15.5-oz.) cans dark beans, flushed and depleted

- 2 c. low-sodium chicken broth, isolated
- 2 tbsp. new lime juice
- 4 cloves garlic, finely chopped
- 1 jalapeño, finely chopped (discretionary)
- 1 (4-oz.) can diced green chile peppers
- 4 c. destroyed rotisserie chicken
- 1/2 c. chopped cilantro takes off, furthermore more for serving
- 8 store-bought tostadas (deep-fried level corn tortillas)
- 3 c. destroyed romaine
- 1 avocado, cut
- 1 c. disintegrated queso fresco or cotija cheese
- Lime wedges, for serving

Headings

Step 1

In a large skillet over medium-high warm, warm 3 tbsp. oil. Include finely chopped onion, cumin, 1 1/2 tsp. salt, and 1 tsp. dark pepper. Cook, stirring occasionally, until onion has relaxed, about 5 minutes. Add beans and 1 c. broth and cook, stirring occasionally, until most fluid has diminished, 5 to 7 minutes. Proceed to cook, employing a potato masher or fork to crush beans, until smooth, 3 to 5 minutes. Evacuate from warm and blend in lime juice.

Step 2

In the meantime, in a medium pot over medium warm, warm remaining 2 tbsp. oil. Include cut onion and remaining 1 1/2 tsp. salt and 1 tsp. dark pepper. Cover and cook, blending sometimes, until onions have relaxed somewhat, 3 to 5 minutes. Include garlic and jalapeño, in case utilizing, and cook, blending, until fragrant, around 1 miniature. Mix in green chiles and remaining 1 c. broth. Increment warm to medium-high and cook, mixing once in a while, until diminished by half, 5-7 minutes. Blend in chicken until warmed through. Remove from warm and mix in cilantro.

Step 3

Beat tostadas with bean blend, chicken blend, romaine, avocado, and queso fresco. Embellish with more cilantro. Serve with lime wedges alongside.

38. Coconut Curry Salmon

This salmon dish can be as zesty as you like it. Fair keep in mind that the coconut drain will tone down a part of the warm so indeed on the off chance that you're feeling just like the called for sum will be as well much, it might not be. The coconut drain and zest go so well together, making a wealthy, but not overwhelming, sauce that truly tastes and feels distant more complicated than it is. The salmon stews within the drain keeping it exceptionally delicate and flaky and of course imparting a lot of flavor onto it. Spoon the sauce over the salmon a couple of times because it cooks to provide it a decent coating and do not disregard to mix the sauce each once in for a short time so nothing begins to burn.

Fixings

- 4 (4-oz.) salmon filets
- Legitimate salt
- Naturally ground dark pepper
- 1 tbsp. vegetable oil
- 1 shallot, meagerly cut
- 1 tbsp. ruddy curry glue
- 2 cloves garlic, minced
- 2 tsp. naturally minced ginger
- 1 (14-oz.) can coconut drain
- 1 tbsp. sriracha
- 1 tbsp. angle sauce
- Cooked rice, for serving
- Lime wedges, for serving

- Crisply chopped cilantro, for serving

Bearings

Step 1

Season salmon with salt and pepper. In a huge skillet over medium warm, warm oil. Include salmon, skin side down and cook until brilliant, approximately 5 minutes per side. Expel from skillet and put on a plate.

Step 2

Return skillet over medium warm and include shallots. Cook until brilliant and delicate, 3 minutes. Include curry glue, garlic, and ginger and cook until glue is obscured and fragrant, 1 miniature. Diminish warm slightly and slowly whisk in coconut drain, at that point include sriracha and angle sauce and bring to a stew. Return salmon to skillet and let stew until pieces effortlessly with a fork and inside temperature comes to 145°, around 15 minutes depending on thickness of salmon. Spoon sauce over salmon and blend sauce every so often. Include more sriracha or angle sauce to taste.

Step 3

Spoon sauce over salmon and present with rice, limes, and finished off with cilantro.

39. Gazpacho with Burrata

Velvety burrata on beat of a tomato and basil gazpacho is the foremost refreshing no-cook summer supper ready to envision. A few gazpacho has bread in it for added texture, but for this adaptation, we preferred the thought of serving toasted bread nearby to plunge into the soup and spread the burrata on. We moreover included a small yogurt to form this additional velvety and for fair a little tang. Be beyond any doubt to blend at a tall speed for a great 2 to 3 minutes to make a silkier gazpacho. You'll be able moreover strain it after mixing to guarantee it's as smooth as conceivable.

Fixings

- 2 lb. tomatoes (such as legacy or Roma), center expelled and quartered
- 2 little seedless cucumbers, quartered
- 1/2 little ruddy onion, cut into wedges
- 1 jalapeño, seeds evacuated
- 1/2 c. pressed basil, additionally more for embellish
- 1/4 c. plain yogurt (ideally whole-milk)
- 2 cloves garlic

- 2 tbsp. ruddy wine vinegar
- Legitimate salt
- Crisply ground dark pepper
- 1/2 c. extra-virgin olive oil, furthermore more for sprinkling
- 8 oz. burrata
- Dried up bread, for serving

Headings

Step 1

In a large food processor or blender, puree tomatoes, cucumbers, onion, jalapeño, basil, yogurt, garlic, and vinegar until smooth; liberally season with salt and dark pepper.

Step 2

With motor running, slowly drizzle in oil. Proceed to mix until smooth, 2 to 3 minutes; season with salt and black pepper to taste.

Step 3

Pour into an expansive bowl or holder and refrigerate until well chilled, around 1 hour.

Step 4

Divide gazpacho among bowls. Cut open burrata and separate among bowls. Sprinkle with more oil and embellish with basil. Serve with bread nearby.

40. Gazpacho with Burrata

Rich burrata on beat of a tomato and basil gazpacho is the foremost refreshing no-cook summer feast able to envision. A few gazpacho has bread in it for included surface, but for this form, we enjoyed the thought of serving toasted bread nearby to plunge into the soup and spread the burrata on. We too included a small yogurt to form this additional velvety and for fair a small tang. Be beyond any doubt to mix at a tall speed for a great 2 to 3 minutes to make a silkier gazpacho. You'll be able to strain it after mixing to guarantee it's as smooth as possible.

Ingredients

- 2 lb. tomatoes (such as legacy or Roma), center evacuated and quartered
- 2 small seedless cucumbers, quartered
- 1/2 little ruddy onion, cut into wedges

- 1 jalapeño, seeds expelled
- 1/2 c. stuffed basil, also more for embellish
- 1/4 c. plain yogurt (preferably whole-milk)
- 2 cloves garlic
- 2 tbsp. ruddy wine vinegar
- Legitimate salt
- Naturally ground dark pepper
- 1/2 c. extra-virgin olive oil, also more for sprinkling
- 8 oz. burrata
- Dried up bread, for serving

Bearings

Step 1

In an expansive nourishment processor or blender, puree tomatoes, cucumbers, onion, jalapeño, basil, yogurt, garlic, and vinegar until smooth; liberally season with salt and dark pepper.

Step 2

With engine running, slowly drizzle in oil. Proceed to mix until smooth, 2 to 3 minutes; season with salt and dark pepper to taste.

Step 3

Pour into a huge bowl or holder and refrigerate until well chilled, about 1 hour.

Step 4

Divide gazpacho among bowls. Cut open burrata and isolate among bowls. Sprinkle with more oil and decorate with basil. Serve with bread alongside.

41. Esquites Corn Chowder

Have you ever had esquites so great, you needed to drink it straight out of the bowl? Esquites is the famous Mexican road nourishment made from corn parts, mayo, lime, and chili powder, like elotes, but in a cup (truly elote en vaso!). When it came to making this soup, I looked no assist than corn chowder the quintessential Unused Britain consolation nourishment that features loads of sweet corn, bacon, and potato. The warm, rich soup and the cool, sweet, acidic esquites combine in one bowl to make a madly great differentiate of surface, temperature, and flavor.

Fixings

- 4 oz. thick-cut bacon, cut into 1/2" pieces
- 4 ears of corn, bits expelled (almost 3 1/2 c.), cobs saved
- 1 tbsp. kosher salt, separated
- 1 tsp. ground epazote (discretionary)
- 1 medium onion, chopped
- 2 jalapeños, seeded and chopped, isolated
- 2 cloves garlic, finely chopped, separated
- 1 enormous reddish brown potato (around 13 oz.), stripped and cleaved into 1/2" pieces
- 4 c. low-sodium vegetable broth
- 1 tsp. chili powder, furthermore more for serving
- 1/2 c. heavy cream
- 2 tbsp. chopped new cilantro
- 2 tbsp. new lime juice
- 2 tbsp. Mexican crema or sour cream
- 1 tbsp. mayonnaise
- 3/4 c. cotija cheese or queso fresco, disintegrated

Bearings

Step 1

In a large Dutch oven or pot over medium warm, cook bacon, mixing, until fresh, 8 to 10 minutes. Deplete and exchange to a plate; reserve bacon fat.

Step 2

In same pot over medium-high warm, warm 2 tbsp. saved fat. Cook corn parts and 1/2 tsp. salt, blending, until corn begins to caramelize, 6 to 7 minutes. Blend in epazote, on the off chance that utilizing. Exchange corn blend to a medium bowl.

Step 3

In same pot over medium-high warm, warm 1 tbsp. saved fat. Cook onion and 1/2 tsp. salt, mixing, until relaxed, almost 2 minutes. Include half of jalapeños and half of garlic and cook, blending, until fragrant, around 1 diminutive more. Mix in potato, broth, chili powder, and 2 tsp. salt. Add corncobs to pot, cover, and cook over medium warm until potatoes are delicate, approximately 15 minutes. Dispose of cobs. Mix soup with a blender, immersion blender, or nourishment processor. Return soup to pot. Cook over moo warm and mix in cream and 2 1/2 c. corn blend.

Step 4

In a little bowl, combine cilantro, lime juice, crema, mayonnaise, and remaining corn blend, jalapeño, and garlic.

Step 5

Divide soup among bowls. Beat with bacon, cilantro blend, cheese, and more chili powder.

42. Garlic Butter Meatballs & Zoodles

Whereas nothing may never supplant the spot pasta holds in our hearts, these garlic butter meatballs and zoodles are an awfully close second. Low-carb and gluten-free, usually a straightforward weeknight supper that will provide on that wealthy pasta sauce taste, whereas making a difference you get in another making a difference of veggies. In our book, that's a supper victor.

Fixings

- 1 lb. ground chicken
- 5 cloves garlic, minced and isolated
- 1 huge egg, beaten

- 1/2 c. naturally ground Parmesan, furthermore more for decorate
- 2 tbsp. naturally chopped parsley
- 1/4 tsp. smashed ruddy pepper pieces
- Legitimate salt
- Crisply ground dark pepper
- 2 tbsp. extra-virgin olive oil
- 4 tbsp. butter
- 1 lb. zoodles
- Juice of 1/2 a lemon

Headings

Step 1

In an expansive bowl, blend ground chicken, 2 cloves garlic (2 teaspoons minced), egg, Parmesan, parsley, and ruddy pepper chips. Season with salt and pepper, at that point frame into tablespoon-size meatballs.

Step 2

In an expansive skillet over medium warm, warm oil and cook meatballs until brilliant on all sides and cooked through, approximately 10 minutes. Exchange to a plate and wipe out skillet with a paper towel.

Step 3

Liquefy butter in skillet and include remaining minced garlic. Cook until fragrant, 1 diminutive. Include zoodles to skillet, hurl with garlic butter, and include lemon juice. Return meatballs to skillet and warm until warmed through.

Step 4

Decorate with Parmesan some time recently serving.

43. Chipotle-Lime Chilaquiles

Fixings

- 2 ears sweet corn
- 2 tbsp. extra-virgin olive oil
- 1/2 sweet onion, diced
- 2 cloves garlic, minced
- 1 medium zucchini, divided longwise and daintily cut
- 2 1/2 c. store-bought ruddy salsa
- 2 tbsp. minced chipotle peppers in adobo sauce
- 1 1/2 c. low-sodium chicken broth
- 14 oz. thick tortilla chips

- Juice and pizzazz of 2 limes
- legitimate salt
- Crisply ground dark pepper
- 1/2 c. queso fresco, disintegrated, for embellish
- 1/2 bunch new cilantro clears out, generally chopped, for embellish
- 1/2 avocado, daintily cut, for embellish
- Lime wedges, for embellish

Bearings

Step 1

Preheat stove to 375°. In a expansive skillet over medium-high warm, include corn and burn, turning cobs each 2 minutes to equally char. Remove corn from skillet and cut bits off every cob, discarding the cobs.

Step 2

Empty oil into skillet and cook onion and garlic, 2 to 3 minutes. Decrease warm to medium and proceed to cook, 2 minutes. Mix in zucchini and cook, 4 to 5 minutes more. Include corn and hurl together. Expel half the blend from skillet and set aside.

Step 3

Include salsa, adobo, and broth and mix together. Bring blend to a bubble and start including tortilla chips, a modest bunch at a time, collapsing delicately to coat each chip. Permit chips to splash up a few fluids some time recently including more. Rehash until all chips have been included and equitably blended.

Step 4

Include lime pizzazz and juice, season with salt and pepper, and delicately overlay together. Prepare until all fluid has been retained, 12 to 15 minutes. Wrap up chilaquiles by topping with remaining zucchini and corn blend, queso fresco, cut avocados, and cilantro. Serve with lime wedges.

44. Stuffed Pepper Casserole

Longing for stuffed peppers with a division of the exertion? Enter:

stuffed pepper casserole. This one-pot ponder packs all the awesome flavor of a stuffed pepper whereas requiring way less effort. We took motivation from our classic stuffed peppers for this casserole, making a blend of ground hamburger, tomato-flavored rice, and melty cheese. That being said, a bit like our other stuffed pepper formulas, you'll be able really explore with this formula to form it your possess. Here's how to form it the leading it can be:

Fixings

- 2 tbsp. extra-virgin olive oil
- 1 lb. (80%) incline ground hamburger
- 2 chime peppers, any color, chopped into 1" pieces
- 1 expansive yellow onion, chopped into 1" pieces
- 3 cloves garlic, daintily cut
- 2 tsp. legitimate salt
- 1 tsp. naturally ground dark pepper
- 1 tsp. ground cumin
- 1 tsp. smoked paprika
- 1/2 tsp. dried oregano
- 1 (6-oz.) can tomato glue
- 1 (14.5-oz.) can fire-roasted diced tomatoes
- 1 1/2 c. meat broth
- 1 c. basmati rice
- 2 c. destroyed pepper Jack cheese (almost 8 oz.)
- 1 tbsp. finely chopped new cilantro

Bearings

Step 1

Preheat stove to 350°. In a huge Dutch stove over medium warm, warm oil. When oil is sparkling, add ground meat and cook, breaking separated with a wooden spoon and mixing once in a while, until cooked through, 4 to 6 minutes.

Step 2

Blend in peppers, onion, garlic, salt, pepper, cumin, paprika, and oregano. Cook, stirring sometimes, until flavors are fragrant, about 1 miniature. Blend in tomato glue and cook, mixing, until fragrant, approximately 2 minutes.

Step 3

Include tomatoes, broth, and rice. Mix until joined, scratching up any browned bits from foot of pot. Increase warm to tall and bring to an air pocket. Promptly cover and exchange to stove. Prepare until rice is delicate, 20 to 24 minutes. Evacuate from broiler and set broiler to tall.

Step 4

Mix once more, at that point beat with cheese. Return to stove, revealed, and broil until cheese is brilliant brown and bubbly, 3 to 4 minutes. Beat with cilantro.

45. Moment Pot Pho

The essential work of an extraordinary soup, other than giving tons of flavor, is to deliver you that warm, stick-to-your-ribs feeling. Few soups do that as well as a piling bowl of pho. The Vietnamese beef-bone based soup is more often than not chock full of noodles, new herbs and any number of garnishes like cilantro, bean grows, meagerly cut circular eye or indeed meatballs. The genuine star, be that as it may, is the broth itself. But, in the event that you inquire any prepared pho-fessional they'll tell you that making a legitimate broth will take you hours, in the event that not an entire day, to develop the wealthy and complex flavors needed for an excellent bowl of the stuff. In the event that you need to undertake to reproduce this broth without the same time investment, one of the leading ways to do usually by employing a weight cooker!

Fixings

FOR BROTH:

- 4 lb. hamburger bones (blend of knuckle and shank)
- 1 cinnamon adhere
- 8 to 10 cloves
- 4 green cardamom or 1 dark cardamom cases
- 2 to 3-star anise cases

- 1 huge onion, peeled and split
- 1 expansive piece ginger (almost 6 ounces), generally chopped
- 4 garlic cloves, crushed
- 2 1/2 tbsp. brown sugar
- 1/3 c. angle sauce
- Legitimate salt
- 1 lb. hamburger brisket or chuck, cut into expansive pieces

FOR Gathering:

- 3/4 lb. flank steak or circular eye
- 1 lb. banh pho noodles (or your #1 rice noodle)
- 1 bunch cilantro, half roughly chopped and half cleared out entire
- Green onions, green parts meagerly cut
- 1 little onion, daintily cut and soaked in cold water for 10 minutes
- Lime wedges
- Bean grows
- Hoisin sauce
- Sriracha

Bearings

FOR BROTH:

Step 1

Fill a huge pot sufficient to cover bones and bring to a rolling boil. Include bones and cook 10 minutes. You should take note a great sum of rubbish and cloudiness in your water. Since the bones are aiming to cook in a weight cooker, there won't be a chance to skim the beat of the broth of the scum, so parboiling the bones makes a difference to diminish cloudiness within the last soup. Strain the bones and wash them beneath cold water, making beyond any doubt to clean absent any remaining scumminess.

Step 2

Set your Moment Pot to sauté. Once the cooker has warmed, include cinnamon, cloves, cardamom, and star anise. Toast flavors for 3 to 4 minutes, until fragrant. Turn off Moment Pot. Include bones, onion, ginger, and garlic to the Moment Pot, at that point cover with 6 glasses of water. Include brown sugar, angle sauce, and a huge squeeze of legitimate salt, and donate it a slight blend to combine. Best everything with the brisket and include fair sufficient water to cover without going over the max pressure line within the Instant Pot.

Step 3

Put the cover on Instant Pot and near it. Move the steam discharge valve to the "sealing position" and set the Moment Pot to "Pressure Cook" on tall for 1 hour. It ought to take 10 to 15 minutes for the weight cooker to seal legitimately.

Step 4

When the soup is done, carefully discharge the steam valve and permit for the Moment Pot to depressurize and for the steam to release. This could take a small whereas, so fair be understanding!

Step 5

When done, set aside the cooked brisket and strain the broth through a fine work strainer into a pot or move the broth to a holder and store within the ice chest for up to 5 days.

Step 6

Discretionary:

For an additional clear, less greasy broth, permit the broth to cool within the fridge for 4 hours or overnight and remove the layer of fat that will have cemented on best of your broth.

FOR Get together:

Step 1

To slice the meat, put within the cooler for 15 to 20 minutes. Remove and cut against the grain as thinly as conceivable. Move the cuts to a place and set aside.

Step 2

Move your banh pho noodles to a huge heatproof bowl and cover with boiling water. Let stand for 15 to 20 minutes or until they have come to your wanted surface. Strain and wash with cold water, set aside. Whereas the noodles are splashing, bring the broth to a bubble in a huge pan.

Step 3

To serve, include some noodles to the foot of each bowl. Include a bit of chopped cilantro, green onion, and onion. Following, include many cuts of the crude hamburger. Cover everything with bubbling broth, which can cook the crude meat. Serve the bowl nearby more cilantro, scallion, and onions, as well as lime wedges, bean grows, hoisin, and sriracha.

46. Arepas

Arepas or cornmeal patties predate the colonization of the Americas and are a prime illustration of innate culinary conventions that remained unaltered by Spanish impact. To a great extent well known in Venezuela, Colombia, and Bolivia, varieties of the arepa are found all through the Latin American world, counting Puerto Rican arepas de coco, Panamanian tortilla changas, Ecuadorian tortillas de maíz, Salvadoran pupusas, and Mexican gorditas.

Fixings

- 2 c. precooked cornmeal (such as Harina P.A.N.)
- 2 tsp. legitimate salt
- 2 1/2 c. warm water
- 2 tbsp. vegetable oil
- 1 (15.5-oz.) can dark beans, depleted, washed, and warmed
- 1 c. destroyed queso blanco or mozzarella
- 1 avocado, daintily cut
- Cilantro takes off, for serving

Step 1

In an expansive bowl, whisk cornmeal and salt to combine Incorporate water and blend in with a wooden spoon until a combination shapes. Cover with a kitchen towel and let hydrate 10 minutes.

Step 2

Isolate mixture into 8 break even with parcels, around 1/2 glass (4 ounces) each. Roll batter into balls, at that point straighten between your palms to a 3"-wide circle almost 1/2" thick.

Step 3

In an expansive cast-iron or nonstick skillet over medium warm, warm 1 tablespoon oil. When oil starts to smoke, include 4 pieces of mixture. Cover skillet and cook until bottoms are pleasantly charred, 5 to 7 minutes. Flip and proceed to cook, revealed, until moment side is charred, 5 to 7 minutes more. Exchange to a plate. Rehash with remaining 1 tablespoon oil and batter.

Step 4

Let cool somewhat, at that point make a take in each arepa by cutting on a level plane almost three-quarters of the way through. Fill pockets with beans, cheese, avocado, and cilantro.

47. Ratatouille Casserole

Ratatouille, a classic conclusion of summer dish from the South of France that highlights our favorite late-season create, takes on a modern frame in this wonderful spiraled casserole. Rather than cooking the ratatouille on the stovetop, appreciate it right out of the broiler, otherwise you can heat the dish ahead of time and let the fixings blend within the fridge overnight for indeed more flavor. Serve with a French dessert at the conclusion to circular out a paramount supper, like our clafoutis or apple tart.

Fixings

- 2 tbsp. dry white wine
- 2 tbsp. tomato glue
- 1 c. diced simmered ruddy chime peppers
- 1/3 c. chopped new basil clears out
- 4 cloves garlic, daintily cut
- Legitimate salt
- Crisply ground dark pepper
- 3 medium Roma tomatoes (almost 3/4 lb. add up to), daintily cut
- 1 huge zucchini (almost 12 oz.), meagerly cut

- 1 little globe eggplant (around 12 oz.), split the long way, meagerly cut into half moons
- 1/3 c. extra-virgin olive oil
- 1 tsp. generally chopped new thyme clears out

Bearings

Step 1

Preheat broiler to 425°. In a shallow 2-quart preparing dish, whisk wine and tomato glue until smooth and combined. Include chime pepper, basil, garlic, 1/4 teaspoon salt, and 1/4 teaspoon pepper. Hurl to combine and spread in an indeed layer.

Step 2

Stack 1 tomato cut, 1 zucchini slice, and 1 eggplant cut and vertically stack along edge of preparing dish, with eggplant skin side confronting up. Rehash with remaining tomato, zucchini, and eggplant cuts, making a winding in preparing dish.

Step 3

Sprinkle vegetables with oil and sprinkle with thyme; season with 3/4 teaspoon salt and a couple of grinds of pepper.

Step 4

Cover preparing dish with thwart and prepare until vegetables are fair beginning to turn delicate and juices are bubbling, almost 30 minutes. Reveal and proceed to heat until vegetables are knife-tender, almost 30 minutes more. Let rest 10 minutes some time recently serving.

Step 5

Make Ahead:

Ratatouille can be heated 1 day ahead. Cover dish with cling wrap and refrigerate.

48. Best-Ever Mexican Tostadas

Tostada shells can be precarious to discover, but we favor to create us possess in any case! Hot and new, there's so much more flavor. Furthermore, the store-bought kind nearly continuously come in a Mammoth bundle in which 50% of them are broken. All that said, these madly velvety beans + quick pickled onions would taste astounding on anything, counting a bundled tostada shell.

Ingredients

- 1/2 little ruddy onion, cut
- Juice of 1 lime
- 2 tbsp. butter
- 2 tbsp. vegetable oil, furthermore more for searing
- 1/2 little yellow onion, minced
- 1/2 tsp. dried oregano
- 1/2 tsp. chili powder
- Legitimate salt
- Crisply ground dark pepper
- 2 (15.5-oz.) cans pinto beans, depleted and flushed
- 6 corn tortillas
- FOR TOPPING
- 1 1/2 c. cotija, disintegrated
- 1 avocado, cut
- 4 radishes, daintily cut into rounds
- 1 jalapeño, daintily cut
- 1/4 c. cilantro clears out
- 1 lime, cut for serving

Headings

Step 1

In a medium bowl, combine ruddy onions and lime juice. Set aside to fast pickle whereas planning the rest of your fixings.

Step 2

In an expansive skillet over medium warm, dissolve butter and warm oil. When oil is hot and butter is frothing, include yellow onion and cook, mixing sometimes, until onions are delicate and translucent, 5 minutes. Include oregano and chili powder and season with salt and pepper and cook until fragrant, 1 miniature more.

Step 3

Include beans and 1/2 glass water. Cook, squashing beans with a wooden spoon or potato masher, until craved consistency is reached. When beans are thick and nearly all water has vanished, expel from warm.

Step 4

In a medium, high-sided skillet, include vegetable oil until it is 1/2" profound. Warm oil until a drop of water sizzles when included to the container. Utilizing tongs, broil 1 tortilla at a time until brilliant and fresh, approximately 20 to 30 seconds per side. Exchange to a paper-towel lined plate and salt quickly.

Step 5

Construct tostadas:

Beat each tortilla with approximately 1/4 glass refried beans, avocado, radishes, jalapeño, cilantro, and a few speedy salted onions. Serve with lime wedges.

49.   Nectar Mustard Chicken

Making a feast in one container may be a fragile dance involving cooking time, temperature, and flavor. One you master that move, you'll see that you just can customize/improvise a bit. Furthermore, doing as few dishes as conceivable may be a joyful feeling.

Fixings

- Legitimate salt
- 2 tbsp. nectar
- 1/4 c. Dijon mustard
- 1 clove garlic, minced or ground
- 1/2 tsp. lime zest
- 1 tbsp. chopped new cilantro clears out, stems saved
- 2 tbsp. extra-virgin olive oil
- 7 oz. Brussels grows, split in case huge

- 1 shallot, peeled and quartered
- 1 1/2 lb
- bone-in, skin-on chicken thighs (around 4 thighs, 6 ounces each)
- 1 little sweet potato, around 7 oz, cut into ½" 3d shapes 1 little
- 1 jalapeño pepper, split the long way, cut into ½" semi circles
- Legitimate salt
- Crisply ground dark pepper

Headings

Step 1

Alter broiler rack to center position and preheat the broiler to 425°.

Step 2

In a medium bowl, whisk until combined nectar, Dijon, garlic, lime pizzazz, 1 tablespoon of cilantro stems, and 1 teaspoon of oil. Exchange half of the dressing to an isolated small bowl. (This will be utilized for the chicken).

Step 3

Include the Brussels grows, shallots, and ½ teaspoon of salt to the remaining dressing within the medium bowl and hurl together so everything is coated.

Step 4

Put each chicken thigh skin-side down on a cutting board, making beyond any doubt to unfurl the abundance folds of skin. Trim the additional skin from around the edge of the meat so that it as it were hangs over around ½". Thoroughly pat each piece dry with a paper towel, and season each piece on both sides with a pinch of salt and a couple of grinds of dark pepper.

Step 5

In an expansive cast press container, warm 1 tablespoon of oil over medium-high warm until the oil gleams. Put the thighs skin-side down, and cook undisturbed for 5 minutes. After 5 minutes, pivot each piece to guarantee the fat is equitably rendered from the skin, and cook for an extra 5 minutes. (The skin ought to be a profound brilliant brown.) Exchange the chicken to a plate. Deplete the fat from the skillet and wipe clean.

Step 6

In a little bowl, combine the sweet potatoes, jalapeños, and remaining teaspoon of oil. Season with many squeezes of salt, and pepper.

Step 7

Return the pan to medium warm and add 1 teaspoon of oil until it shines.

Step 8

Orchestrate the vegetables within the dish so that the Brussels grows are confront down around the exterior edge. Another, make a ring of the sweet potatoes and jalapeño. At long last, orchestrate shallots, cut-side down, in the center. Place the chicken thighs on beat of the sweet potatoes, jalapeño, and shallots, skin side up. Maintain a strategic distance from covering the outer layer of Brussels grows to assist keep them from steaming and getting as well mushy.

Step 9

Exchange the skillet to the broiler, and cook for 15 minutes, The Brussels grows ought to have a profound brown coloring on their cut surface. Evacuate container from the broiler and brush the tops of the chicken thighs with remaining dressing. (For additional fresh skin, brush the marinade on the underside of each piece of chicken rather than on beat.) Broil for an extra 5 minutes, evacuate from the broiler, and beat with chopped cilantro

50. Heated Risotto with Lemon, Peas & Parmesan

Some dishes immediately summon up dreams of long, romantic dinners in Italy. There's sheep ragù, veal marsala, and of course, perfectly velvety risotto. Thankfully, you do not get to get on a plane to eat it, or indeed go out to an eatery. It's all conceivable with this heated risotto with lemon, peas, and Parmesan.

Fixings

- 4 tbsp. butter
- 1 lemon
- 1 yellow onion, finely chopped
- 2 cloves garlic, finely chopped
- 1 c. Arborio rice
- 3 1/2 c. chicken or vegetable broth
- 1 1/2 tsp. kosher salt
- 1/2 c. ground Parmesan (2 oz.), also more for serving
- 1 c. solidified peas, defrosted
- 1/2 tsp. naturally ground dark pepper
- Chopped new parsley, for embellish

Headings

Step 1

Preheat broiler to 375°F. Liquefy 2 tablespoons butter in a Dutch broiler over medium-high warm.

Step 2

Employing a Y-peeler, expel two 1"-thick strips of zest from the lemon. Include onion and lemon pizzazz to the butter and cook, mixing regularly, until mellowed, around 5 minutes. Include garlic and Incorporate garlic and cook, blending, until fragrant, around 1 modest. Mix in rice, broth, and 1 teaspoon salt. Bring to a simmer, cover, and transfer to the broiler.

Step 3

Bake until rice is delicate, 20 minutes. Carefully remove the top and stir in Parmesan, peas, pepper, remaining 2 tablespoons butter and ½ teaspoon salt, blending until butter is softened and peas are warm. Cut the lemon in half and press half of the juice into the risotto; blend to combine. Remove lemon pizzazz and serve topped with more Parmesan and parsley.

51. Butternut Squash Curry

Sometime recently we handle anything else, let's center on the well-known term we all know as curry, a nourishment gather that may be classified as its possess with different implications and formulas around the world. Curry frequently alludes to the blend of seasonings and a stew made with vegetables, meat, and parcels of flavors. From India to China, Japan, and Jamaica, the thought of what "curry" implies has certainly advanced.

Fixings

- 1 expansive butternut squash (around 2 1/2 lb.), peeled, seeded, and cut into huge chunks
- 5 tbsp. impartial oil, isolated
- Legitimate salt
- 1 huge ruddy onion, coarsely chopped
- 5 cloves garlic, minced
- 2 tbsp. curry powder
- 2 (13.5-oz.) cans full-fat coconut drain
- 1 huge bunch of wavy kale (approximately 6.5 oz.), generally chopped
- Juice of 1 lime
- 1/4 c. chopped new parsley
- 1/4 c. sunflower seeds

- Cooked rice, for serving

Headings

Step 1

Preheat stove to 400°. In a huge bowl, blend squash with 3 tablespoons oil; season with salt. On a rimmed heating sheet, orchestrate squash in an indeed layer. Cook until delicate and brilliant brown, 35 to 40 minutes.

Step 2

In the interim, in an expansive skillet over medium-high heat, heat remaining 2 tablespoons oil. Include onion, season with salt, and cook, mixing every so often, until softly brilliant, 8 minutes. Decrease warm to medium-low. Incorporate garlic and cook, blending, until fragrant, around 1 smaller than normal. Include curry powder and cook, mixing, until combined. Increment warm to medium and include coconut drain. Bring to a stew, at that point include kale; season with salt. Cook, mixing sometimes, until delicate and shriveled, almost 3 minutes. Expel from warm until squash wraps up simmering.

Step 3

Include squash and lime juice to skillet and mix to combine.

Step 4

Separate rice among bowls. Spoon squash blend over, at that point best with parsley and sunflower seeds.

Step 5

Make Ahead:

Squash can be simmered 1 day ahead. Let cool, at that point exchange to a waterproof holder and chill.

52.   Coconut Curry Shrimp & Peas

Say farewell to ho-hum weeknight suppers. This coconut curry shrimp and peas formula could be a fast course to a scrumptious, crowd-pleasing supper. You'll begin by building up flavor with a blend of onion, new ginger, garlic, and serrano chiles. Following, a sprinkling of spices garam masala, paprika, and turmeric infuses the coconut drain. All that's cleared out to do is poach the shrimp specifically within the broth and warm the peas and spinach through, and you're prepared for supper. Served spooned over brown rice or white rice, typically a fast, simple supper that will gain a spot on the customary weeknight turn.

Fixings

- 1 tbsp. virgin coconut or vegetable oil
- 1 little yellow onion, finely chopped
- 1 (2") piece ginger, stripped, finely cleaved (around 1 tbsp.)
- 1/2 serrano chile, exceptionally daintily cut, seeds evacuated in case craved for less warm
- 4 cloves garlic, finely chopped
- Legitimate salt
- 2 tbsp. tomato glue
- 2 tsp. garam masala
- 2 tsp. sweet paprika
- 1 tsp. ground turmeric
- 1 (14-oz.) can full-fat coconut drain
- 1 tsp. brown sugar
- 1 1/2 lb. large (16/20) shrimp, peeled, deveined
- 1 (10-oz.) pack solidified petite peas (about 2 c.)
- 5 oz. infant spinach
- 2 tbsp. new lime juice
- Cooked white or brown rice and lime wedges, for serving

Step 1

In an expansive skillet over medium-high warm, warm oil. Include onion, ginger, Chile, garlic, and 1/4 teaspoon salt. Cook, mixing habitually, until onion is translucent and ginger and garlic are fragrant, 3 to 5 minutes.

Step 2

Include tomato glue, garam masala, paprika, and turmeric and cook, mixing, until fragrant, around 1 diminutive. Include coconut drain, brown sugar, and 1/4 teaspoon salt; bring to a stew. Include shrimp and cook, hurling shrimp a couple of times, unthank of burrata serving of mixed greens as the classic caprese salad's favor cousin. We best peak-summer tomatoes with tasty burrata cheese, and embellish with a shower of peppery basil takes off and savory chives. In the event that you've never had burrata, envision a shell of mozzarella filled with a delicate, rich filling (persuaded however?). It sets flawlessly with the sweet, succulent tomatoes, making this the culminate reviving summer serving of mixed greens to appreciate all season long. Read on for all of our top recommendations on how to form it the finest. I almost cooked through, 3 to 5 minutes. Include peas and spinach and cook, hurling, until spinach is shriveled, peas are warmed, and shrimp is cooked through, almost 2 minutes more. Blend in lime juice; season with more salt, on the off chance that required.

Step 3

Separate rice among bowls. Beat with shrimp blend. Serve with lime wedges nearby.

53. Burrata Serving of mixed greens

Think of burrata salad as the classic caprese salad's favor cousin. We best peak-summer tomatoes with delectable burrata cheese, and embellish with a shower of peppery basil clears out and savory chives. In the event that you've never had burrata, envision a shell of mozzarella filled with a delicate, rich filling (persuaded however?). It pairs perfectly with the sweet, delicious tomatoes, making this the idealize reviving summer serving of mixed greens to appreciate all season long. Examined on for all of our beat tips about how to form it the leading.

Fixings

- 3 lb. legacy or beefsteak tomatoes (almost 4 huge), cut into 1/2" rounds
- 1 shallot, finely chopped
- Flaky ocean salt
- Naturally ground black pepper
- 2 tbsp. extra-virgin olive oil

- 2 tbsp. ruddy wine vinegar
- 1/3 c. panko bread pieces
- 2 (4-oz.) balls burrata, depleted and room temperature
- 1 tbsp. chopped new basil
- 1 tbsp. cut new chives
- Dried up bread, for serving
- Bearings
- Step 1

On a rimmed preparing sheet, hurl tomatoes and shallot; season with 1 teaspoon salt and 1 teaspoon pepper. Sprinkle oil and vinegar over. Let sit until tomatoes have discharged their fluid and shallots are mollified, approximately 30 minutes.

Step 2

In a little skillet over moo warm, toast panko, mixing sometimes, until brilliant brown, around 2 minutes. Exchange to a little bowl.

Step 3

Layer tomatoes on an expansive platter. Spoon shallot and juices over best. Sprinkle with panko. Organize burrata in center of tomatoes and split open together with your hands. Sprinkle with basil, chives, salt, and pepper. Serve with bread nearby.

54. Broiled Chickpea and Avocado Serving of mixed greens

We cherish a healthy, studded serving of mixed greens with a great dressing, and this one is fair that. Chickpeas get simmered plain so that they have a genuine chance to dry and gotten to be extra crispy. In case you've got a discuss fryer, use it to cook your chickpeas for the extreme crisp. The tahini farm could be a lightened-up dressing that's superior than any bottle you may purchase and makes this entirety serving of mixed greens meal-worthy. It's a idealize summer serving of mixed greens for lunch or an excursion!

Fixings

CHICKPEAS

- 1 (15-oz.) can chickpeas, flushed and drained1
- tbsp. extra-virgin olive oil
- 1 tsp. chili powder
- 1/2 tsp. garlic powder
- Kosher salt
- Naturally ground dark pepper

DRESSING

- 1/4 c. plain Greek yogurt (ideally whole-fat)

- 1/4 c. tahini
- Juice of 1 lemon
- 1 tbsp. Dijon mustard
- 1/4 c. (or more) warm water
- 2 tbsp. naturally chopped parsley
- 2 tbsp. sliced chives
- Legitimate salt
- Naturally ground dark pepper
- Squeeze of smashed ruddy pepper chips
- Serving of mixed greens
- 2 heads of romaine, chopped
- 1/2 red onion, meagerly sliced
- 1 avocado, finely chopped
- 1 c. divided cherry tomatoes
- 4 oz. disintegrated feta

Bearings

CHICKPEAS

Step 1

Preheat stove to 400°. Pat chickpeas dry with paper towels and organize in a single layer on a small baking sheet.

Step 2

Broil chickpeas until brilliant and dried out, around 35 minutes.

Step 3

Exchange chickpeas to a medium bowl. Include oil, chili powder, and garlic powder and hurl to combine; season with salt and dark pepper.

DRESSING

Step 1

In a medium bowl, mix yogurt, tahini, lemon juice, and mustard. Stir in warm water, including more water 1 tablespoon at a time on the off chance that required to extricate dressing to a pourable consistency.

Step 2

Include parsley and chives; season with salt, dark pepper, and ruddy pepper pieces and mix to combine.

Serving of mixed greens

In an expansive bowl, put romaine. Beat with onion, avocado, tomatoes, feta, and chickpeas. Sprinkle with dressing and hurl to combine.

55. Dark Bean Tostadas

During busy weeknights, we can't get sufficient of quick, simple, and cheap meals. With only 5 fixings and less than 30 minutes, these dark bean tostadas will have you serving up a straightforward and scrumptious vegan supper on the table with barely any work at all. These tostadas utilize fixings you're more than likely to have on hand, making them the easiest last-minute feast to throw together when you just can't be bothered to cook up anything else. The best part? Since of their effortlessness, these tostadas are perpetually versatile. Make them as-is for the foremost essential form, or utilize them as a base to include all your favorite seasonings and garnishes.

Fixings

- 2 (15-oz.) cans dark beans, washed and depleted
- 8 tostadas
- 2 c. destroyed pepper jack
- Avocado, cut
- Hot sauce

Bearings

Step 1

Preheat stove to 350°. In a little pot over medium warm, include beans and 1 glass of water. Bring to a stew and let stew until beans are warmed through, approximately 10 minutes. Crush with a wooden spoon until most of the beans are crushed with a few entire remaining. Include more water as required to assist make a smoother consistency.

Step 2

In the meantime, put tostadas on an expansive heating sheet and sprinkle cheese equitably over each. Heat until cheese is melty, approximately 5 minutes.

Step 3

Beat tostadas with beans, avocado cuts, and hot sauce.

56. Zucchini Cross Section Lasagna

Beyond any doubt, classic lasagna is delightful. In some cases, in spite of the fact that, we need something a tad less carb-heavy. This zucchini cross section lasagna is the culminate way to help up the classic dish for summer. Master tip:

Zucchini discharges a great sum of water, so we like to spot it with a paper towel when the lasagna is done cooking, and after that broil until the cheese is bubbly and fresh.

Fixings

- 2 c. ricotta
- 1 c. crisply ground Parmesan, furthermore more for sprinkling
- 2 huge eggs
- Legitimate salt
- Crisply ground dark pepper
- 1 1/2 c. marinara sauce
- 3 expansive zucchinis, cut into wide strips employing a Y peeler and depleted on paper towels
- 3 c. destroyed mozzarella

Bearings

Step 1

Preheat stove to 350°. In a little bowl, blend together ricotta, Parmesan, and eggs and season blend with salt and pepper.

Step 2

Spread a lean layer of marinara in a preparing dish. Cover with 2 layers of zucchini, 33% of the ricotta mix, and 33% of the mozzarella. Spread approximately 1/3 container marinara over mozzarella. Rehash layering twice more.

Step 3

For the best, layer zucchini noodles side by side on an inclining within the preparing dish to form a cross section. Lift the foot half of each other noodle and lay another zucchini noodle over askew. Rehash until full.

Step 4

Sprinkle with additional Parmesan and season with salt and pepper.

Step 5

Prepare until melty and zucchini is cooked through, 30 minutes.

Step 6

Let rest for 10 minutes some time recently cutting.

57. Slow-Cooker Ruddy Wine Meat Stew

In case you would like a pardon to induce your moderate cooker out, usually it! Stewing hamburger, potatoes, tomatoes, and onions together for hours makes one of the foremost deeply fulfilling stews you'll ever eat. And while rosemary and sun-dried tomatoes may not be conventional, we think they punch up the flavor and allow a fun bend. This is often consolation nourishment at its best, so dish up a bowl, twist up on the lounge chair with a spoon, and you're completely SET.

Fixings

- 3 lb. hamburger chuck, cut into 2" pieces
- Kosher salt
- Crisply ground black pepper
- 2 tbsp. extra-virgin olive oil
- 2 tbsp. butter
- 1 2/3 c. dry ruddy wine
- 1 tbsp. tomato glue
- 2 Yukon Gold potatoes, cut into 1" 3d shapes
- 3 carrots, chopped into 1" pieces
- 3 celery stalks, chopped into 1" pieces
- 2 onions, chopped into quarters
- 1 c. chopped sun-dried tomatoes
- 4 cloves garlic, minced
- 1 expansive rosemary sprig

- 2 c. low-sodium meat broth
- 1 (28-oz.) can pulverized tomatoes
- Crisply chopped parsley, for embellish

Bearings

Step 1

In a large blending bowl, pat beef dry with a paper towel. Season liberally with salt and pepper.

Step 2

In an expansive skillet over medium-high warm, warm oil. Burn meat on all sides until brilliant brown with a hull, working in clumps in the event that fundamental, almost 10 minutes. Transfer meat to moderate cooker.

Step 3

Include butter and rub container with a wooden spoon to release all browned meat bits. Mix in ruddy wine and tomato glue; stew for 1 diminutive, at that point exchange to moderate cooker.

Step 4

Incorporate potatoes, carrots, celery, onions, sun-dried tomatoes, garlic, rosemary, meat stock, and crushed tomatoes to direct cooker. Season with salt and cook on tall until meat is delicate, 4 to 5 hours.

Step 5

Expel stalk of rosemary. Embellish with parsley some time recently serving.

58. Zucchini Lasagna Roll-Ups

This formula takes a few time and persistence, but it's almost the prettiest "pasta" dish you'll ever see. On the off chance that you have got mandolin, utilize it to form the noodles; in the event that you do not, hone your cut skills.

Fixings

- 6 large zucchini
- 1 (16-oz.) container ricotta
- 3/4 c. naturally grated Parmesan, separated
- 2 expansive eggs
- 1/2 tsp. garlic powder

- Legitimate salt
- Crisply ground dark pepper
- 1 c. marinara
- 1 c. ground mozzarella

Headings

Step 1

Preheat broiler to 400°. Cut zucchini the long way into ⅛" thick strips, at that point put strips on a paper towel-lined preparing sheet to deplete.

Step 2

Make ricotta blend:

In a little bowl, combine ricotta, 1/2 glass Parmesan, eggs, and garlic powder, and season with salt and pepper.

Step 3

Spread a lean layer of marinara onto the foot of a 9"-x-13" baking dish. On each slice of zucchini, spoon a lean layer of sauce, spread ricotta blend on beat, and sprinkle with mozzarella. Roll up and put in preparing dish, pressed together firmly.

Step 4

Sprinkle with remaining 1/4 glass Parmesan. Prepare until zucchini is tender and cheese is melty, 20 minutes.

Budget-Friendly Gluten-Free Suppers

59.   Herb-Grilled Chicken Frites

We join new spices, escapades, lemon juice and olive oil close to the juices gathered from the chicken since it rests to frame a fundamental sauce that perks up this take on poulet frites, or chicken and fries.

Fixings

- 1 ¾ pounds bone-in, skin-on chicken thighs¾
- teaspoon salt, partitioned
- ¾ teaspoon ground pepper, separated
- 5 tablespoons extra-virgin olive oil, isolated
- 2 tablespoons lemon juice

- 1 ½ mugs chopped new herbs, such as basil, parsley, chives and/or oregano
- 1 ½ pounds chestnut potatoes, cut into wedges
- ¼ glass capers, flushed
- ¼ container washed cured jalapeños

Headings

Step 1

Preheat flame broil to medium-high.

Step 2

Sprinkle chicken with 1/2 teaspoon each salt and pepper.

Whisk 2 tablespoons oil, lemon juice and spices in a medium bowl. Save 1/2 glass for sauce, at that point include the chicken to the bowl and rub the remaining herb blend onto it. Let stand for 5 minutes.

Step 3

Hurl potatoes with 1 tablespoon oil and the remaining 1/4 teaspoon each salt and pepper. Flame broil the potatoes and chicken, flipping every so often, until the potatoes are browned and delicate, approximately 15 minutes, and the chicken is crispy and an instant-read thermometer embedded within the thickest portion registers 165 degrees F, 15 to 20 minutes.

Step 4

Exchange the potatoes to a serving platter and tent with thwart to keep warm. Exchange the chicken to a clean cutting board and tent with thwart. Let rest for 5 minutes, at that point include to the platter.

Step 5

Incorporate the saved spice mix, tricks, jalapeños and the leftover 2 tablespoons oil to the juices on the cutting board. Chop the blend into a glue and spread over the chicken.

60. Skillet Buffalo Chicken

In the event that you like Buffalo wings, you'll cherish this speedy skillet Buffalo chicken formula. Chicken cutlets are sautéed, at that point covered in a creamy-spicy sauce. A side-salad embellish of carrots, celery and blue cheese pulls it all together.

Fixings

- 1-pound chicken cutlets
- ¼ teaspoon salt, partitioned
- ¼ teaspoon ground pepper, partitioned
- 1 tablespoon extra-virgin olive oil
- ½ glass finely chopped onion

- ¼ container white wine or low-sodium chicken broth
- ¼ cup hot sauce, for example, Straight to the point's Super hot½
- container heavy cream
- ½ container finely diced carrots
- ⅓ container finely diced celery
- 2 tablespoons disintegrated blue cheese

Bearings

Step 1

Sprinkle chicken with 1/8 teaspoon salt and 1/8 teaspoon pepper. Warm oil in an expansive skillet over medium warm. Include the chicken and cook, turning once, until browned and an instant-read thermometer embedded into the thickest portion registers 165 degrees F, approximately 6 minutes. Exchange to a plate.

Step 2

Include onion to the dish. Cook, mixing, for 1 miniature. Include wine (or broth) and hot sauce; cook, scratching up any browned bits, until the fluid has diminished by half, almost 2 minutes. Blend in cream, any collected juices from the chicken and the remaining 1/8 teaspoon each salt and pepper; stew for 2 minutes. Return the chicken to the dish and turn to coat with the sauce.

Hurl carrots, celery and blue cheese together in a little bowl. Serve chicken topped with the sauce, with the carrot blend on the side.

61. Ancient Bay Salmon with Lemony Squashed Peas

Cooking butter until it browns includes a toasty, nutty flavor to this simple skillet salmon formula. Here it gives Ancient Bay-rubbed salmon a chef-worthy finish—not awful for 20 minutes!

Fixings

- 1 pound peas, new or solidified
- ¼ glass crème fraîche or acrid cream
- ½ teaspoon lemon pizzazz
- 3 tablespoons lemon juice
- ¼ teaspoon salt
- ¼ teaspoon ground pepper
- 1 tablespoon extra-virgin olive oil

- 1 ¼ pounds skin-on salmon, cut into 4 pieces
- 2 teaspoons Ancient Inlet flavoring
- 1 tablespoon butter
- 2 teaspoons new thyme takes off
- Lemon wedges for serving

Headings

Step 1

Bring a medium pot of water to a bubble over tall warm. Include peas and cook until delicate, approximately 5 minutes. Save 1/4 glass of the water, then drain. Combine the peas, the saved water, crème fraiche (or acrid cream), lemon pizzazz, lemon juice, salt and pepper in a nourishment processor. Beat until generally chopped. Spread onto a serving platter.

Step 2

Warm oil in a huge cast-iron or nonstick skillet over medium-high warm. Sprinkle salmon with Ancient Narrows and include to the dish, skin-side up. Cook, flipping once, until it is browned and chips with a fork, 6 to 7 minutes add up to.

Step 3

Orchestrate the salmon on beat of the peas. Include butter and thyme to the container. Cook, mixing, until the butter is brown and fragrant, approximately 30 seconds. Sprinkle over the salmon. Serve with lemon wedges, in case wanted.

62. Dark Bean-Cauliflower "Rice" Bowl

This fragrant cauliflower rice bowl comes together in minutes and could be a straightforward meal for one. Using frozen riced cauliflower rather than rice decreases the carb content—and makes for faster prep.

Fixings

- 1 tablespoon olive oil also 2 tsp., separated
- 1 container solidified cauliflower rice
- ⅛ teaspoon salt
- 2 tablespoons chopped onion
- 2 tablespoons chopped green chime pepper
- ½ teaspoon chili powder
- ½ teaspoon ground cumin
- ¼ teaspoon dried oregano

- ⅔ glass no-salt-added canned dark beans, washed
- 2 tablespoons chopped broiled ruddy pepper
- ¼ container water
- 1 tablespoon lime juice
- ¼ glass shredded reduced-fat Cheddar cheese
- 1 medium tomato, chopped
- 1 tablespoon cleaved new cilantro for finish

Headings

Step 1

Warm 1 Tbsp. oil in a medium skillet over medium warm. Include cauliflower rice and salt; cook, mixing regularly, until warmed through, 3 to 5 minutes. Exchange to a small bowl and keep warm. Wipe out the pan.

Step 2

Warm the remaining 2 tsp. oil within the skillet over medium warm. Include onion, green pepper, chili powder, cumin, and oregano; cook, mixing regularly, until the vegetables are mollified, around 3 minutes. Include beans, simmered ruddy pepper, and water; bring to a simmer. Cook, blending every so often, until warmed through and thickened, 3 to 5 minutes. Evacuate from warm. Mix in lime juice.

Step 3

Orchestrate the bean blend with the hot cauliflower rice in a super bowl. Best with cheese and tomato. Decorate with cilantro, on the off chance that craved.

63.   Gluten-Free Teriyaki Chicken with Broccoli

Everybody loves teriyaki chicken and this one is way better for you with much less included sugar. It's too gluten-free so long as you utilize tamari (aka gluten-free soy sauce). Go ahead and trade out the broccoli for any veggie carrots, snow peas, green beans that you have available.

Fixings

- 1 tablespoon grapeseed oil
- 1 pound boneless, skinless chicken bosoms, cut into 1-inch pieces
- 3 glasses new broccoli florets (8 oz.)
- ¼ container lower-sodium tamari
- 2 tablespoons pineapple juice
- 1 ½ tablespoons honey
- 1 tablespoon rice vinegar
- 2 teaspoons ground garlic

- 2 teaspoons cornstarch
- 1 teaspoon ground new ginger
- 2 (8.8 ounce) pockets precooked microwaveable brown rice, arranged concurring to bundle directions
- ¼ glass meagerly cut scallions
- 1 teaspoon toasted sesame seeds

Directions

Step 1

Warm oil in a huge skillet over tall warm. Include chicken; cook, mixing regularly, until browned and generally cooked, almost 6 minutes. Add broccoli; cook, mixing frequently, until shinning green and delicate, almost 5 minutes.

Step 2

In the meantime, stir together tamari, pineapple juice, honey, vinegar, garlic, cornstarch and ginger in a little bowl.

Step 3

Include the tamari blend to the chicken blend within the dish. Cook over tall warm, mixing continually, until the fluid is thickened and the blend is coated, around 20 seconds. Remove from warm. Serve the chicken blend over rice; sprinkle evenly with scallions and sesame seeds.

64.   64. Stuffed Warmed Potatoes with Pesto& Eggs

Beat prepared potatoes with fried eggs, pesto, spinach and bacon for a stacked heated potato that's idealize for a straightforward supper or generous brunch. Overlook the bacon for a veggie lover form that's fair as scrumptious.

Fixings

4 medium reddish brown potatoes (almost 8 ounces each)

½ cup pesto

2 cups sautéed spinach (see Related Formulas)

4 expansive eggs, browned or poached

4 teaspoons disintegrated cooked bacon

Headings

Step 1

Penetrate potatoes all over with a fork. Microwave on Medium, turning once or twice, until delicate, around 20 minutes. (On the other hand, heat potatoes at 425 degrees F until tender, 45 minutes to 1 hour.) Exchange to a clean cutting board and let cool marginally.

Step 2

Holding them with a kitchen towel to ensure your hands, make a longwise cut to open the potato, but do not cut all the way through. Pinch the ends to uncover the tissue.

Top each potato with a few pesto, spinach, an egg and bacon. Serve warm.

Solid Soup Formulas

65.   Slow-Cooker Spiced Lentil Soup with Vegetables

Flavors frequently utilized in Moroccan food like turmeric, cumin, cinnamon and dark pepper donate this soup complexity and profound flavor. Make it a day ahead, in the event that you'll, to provide the flavors time to blend and create. This simple slow-cooker recipe makes it a cinch to urge the soup cooking whereas you are doing other things.

Fixings

- 2 mugs chopped onions
- 2 mugs chopped carrots
- 4 cloves garlic, minced
- 2 teaspoons extra-virgin olive oil
- 1 teaspoon ground cumin
- 1 teaspoon ground coriander
- 1 teaspoon ground turmeric
- ¼ teaspoon ground cinnamon
- ¼ teaspoon ground pepper
- 6 mugs vegetable broth or reduced-sodium chicken broth
- 2 glasses water
- 3 mugs chopped cauliflower
- 1 ¾ mugs dried green lentils
- 1 (28 ounce) can diced tomatoes
- 2 tablespoons tomato glue
- 4 mugs chopped new spinach or one (10 ounce) bundle solidified chopped spinach, defrosted
- ½ glass chopped new cilantro

- 2 tablespoons lemon juice

Heading

Step 1

Combine onions, carrots, garlic, oil, cumin, coriander, turmeric, cinnamon and pepper in a 5- to 6-quart moderate cooker (see Tip).

Step 2

Include broth, water, cauliflower, lentils, tomatoes and tomato glue and blend until well combined.

Step 3

Cover and cook until the lentils are delicate, 4 to 5 hours on Tall or 8 to 10 hours on Moo.

Step 4

Amid the final 30 minutes of cooking, blend in spinach. Fair some time recently serving, stir in cilantro and lemon juice.

66. Tinola (Filipino Ginger-Garlic Chicken Soup)

Tinola, a comforting Filipino soup prepared with bounty of ginger and garlic, has incalculable varieties all through the Philippines. The soup calls for malunggay takes off (aka moringa), which can be found new or solidified at Asian markets. Bok choy may be a good substitute. Feel free to increment the sums of garlic and angle sauce for an indeed more flavorful soup. Serve this easy and solid chicken soup on its own or with jasmine rice, quinoa or wild rice.

Fixings

- 3 tablespoons canola oil or avocado oil
- ½ glass chopped yellow onion
- ¼ container daintily cut new ginger
- 6 cloves garlic, minced
- 1 pound boneless, skinless chicken thighs, trimmed and cut into 1/2-inch pieces
- 4 mugs low-sodium chicken broth
- 1 ½ mugs peeled and cubed green papaya or chayote
- 2 glasses chopped malunggay takes off or bok choy takes off

- 1 tablespoon angle sauce
- ¼ teaspoon salt
- ¼ teaspoon ground dark pepper

Bearings

Warm oil in a huge pot over medium warm. Include onion, ginger and garlic; cook, blending, until the onion begins to turn translucent, approximately 3 minutes. Add chicken and broth; cook, stirring, until the chicken is just cooked through, almost 5 minutes. Include papaya (or chayote), malunggay (or bok choy), angle sauce, salt and pepper; proceed simmering until the vegetables are delicate and the flavors have melded, almost 5 minutes more.

67. Chunky Cheeseburger Soup

A spoonful of this tomatoes cheeseburger soup conveys the encounter of an idealize burger bite--savory meat and onions, sweet and tart condiments and, of course, Cheddar and American cheese! This kid-friendly and simple soup is beyond any doubt to offer to everybody in your family.

Ingredients

- 1 pound 90%-lean ground meat
- 1 glass chopped celery
- ½ container diced onion
- 4 mugs low-sodium hamburger broth
- 1 glass water
- 4 glasses diced peeled potatoes
- 4 tablespoons unsalted butter (1/2 adhere)
- ¼ glass all-purpose flour
- 1 ½ glasses low-fat milk
- 1 (6 ounce) can no-salt-added tomato glue
- 2 tablespoons ketchup
- 2 tablespoons Dijon mustard
- 2 glasses destroyed Cheddar & American cheese blend
- 1 tablespoon chopped fresh parsley
- Chopped tomatoes, onion and/or dill pickles for decorate

Bearings

Step 1

Cook meat in an expansive pot over medium-high warm, disintegrating with a wooden spoon, until not pink, approximately 5 minutes. Include celery and onion; cook, blending, until the vegetables are mellowed, almost 3 minutes. Include broth, water and potatoes. Bring to a bubble. Diminish warm to a stew, in part cover and cook, mixing every so often, until the potatoes are delicate, around 15 minutes.

Step 2

In the interim, dissolve butter in a medium pot over medium warm. Whisk in flour. Gradually include drain, blending always, and cook until thickened, approximately 2 minutes. Whisk in tomato paste, ketchup and mustard.

Step 3

Gradually whisk the drain blend into the soup and bring to a bubble. Diminish warm to a stew and mix in cheese, a modest bunch at a time. Cook fair until the cheese is softened. Expel from warm and blend in parsley. Serve topped with tomatoes, onion and/or pickles, if desired.

68.   Classic Chicken Soup

Classic chicken noodle soup gets a sound overhaul with low-sodium chicken broth, whole-wheat egg noodles and tons of vegetables. To induce a homemade stock flavor using store-bought broth, we simmer bone-in chicken breasts within the broth some time recently including the rest of the soup ingredients. But you're brief on time, feel free to utilize pre-cooked chicken and begin the formula at step 2.

Fixings

- 2 tablespoons extra-virgin olive oil
- 1 container chopped onion
- 2 large cloves garlic, minced
- 1 tablespoon chopped new thyme or 1 teaspoon dried
- 1 cove leaf
- 8 mugs low-sodium chicken broth
- 2 pounds' bone-in chicken breasts, skin evacuated
- 2 mugs cut celery
- 2 mugs cut carrots
- 2 glasses frozen peas
- 1 ¼ teaspoons salt
- ½ teaspoon ground pepper
- 3 glasses cooked whole-wheat egg noodles
- ¼ container chopped new parsley

Bearings

Step 1

Warm oil in an expansive pot over medium warm. Include onion and garlic and cook, stirring occasionally, until mellowed, 2 to 3 minutes. Add thyme and cove leaf; cook, blending, for 1 miniature. Include broth and chicken. Cover, increment warm to tall and bring to a simmer. Uncover and cook, turning the chicken every so often, until an instant-read thermometer embedded into the thickest portion without touching bone registers 165 degrees F, 20 to 22 minutes. Skim any froth from the surface as the chicken cooks. Transfer the chicken to a clean cutting board. When cool sufficient to handle, expel the meat from the bones and shred.

Step 2

In the meantime, include celery, carrots and peas to the pot; return to a stew. Cook until the vegetables are delicate, 4 to 10 minutes. Blend within the shredded chicken, salt, pepper and noodles and cook until warmed through, approximately 3 minutes more. Evacuate from warm and mix in parsley.

69. Sweet Potato-Peanut Bisque

This fulfilling veggie lover sweet potato soup is motivated by the flavors of West African shelled nut soup. We just like the added zip of hot green chiles, but they can some of the time be very zesty. It's best to require a little chomp first and add them to taste. Try chopped peanuts and scallions for a distinctive garnish. Serve with a blended green serving of mixed greens with vinaigrette.

Fixings

- 2 expansive sweet potatoes (10-12 ounces each)
- 1 tablespoon canola oil
- 1 little yellow onion, chopped
- 1 expansive clove garlic, minced
- 3 mugs reduced-sodium tomato-vegetable juice mix or tomato juice
- 1 (4 ounce) can diced green chiles, ideally hot, depleted
- 2 teaspoons minced new ginger
- 1 teaspoon ground allspice
- 1 (15 ounce) can vegetable broth
- ½ glass smooth common shelled nut butter
- Naturally ground pepper to taste

- Chopped new cilantro leaves for embellish

Bearings

Step 1

Prick sweet potatoes in a few places with a fork. Microwave on High until just cooked through, 7 to 10 minutes. Set aside to cool.

Step 2

Meanwhile, warm oil in an expansive pot or Dutch stove over medium-high warm. Include onion and cook, stirring, until it fair starts to brown, 2 to 4 minutes. Add garlic and cook, blending, for 1 miniature more. Mix in juice, green chiles, ginger and allspice. Alter the warm so the mixture bubbles delicately; cook for 10 minutes.

Step 3

In the interim, peel the sweet potatoes and chop into bite-size pieces. Include half to the pot. Put the other half in a food processor or blender together with broth and shelled nut butter. Puree until totally smooth. Include the puree to the pot and mix well to combine. Lean the bisque with water, in case wanted. Season with pepper. Warm until hot. Embellish with cilantro, in the event that wanted.

70. Petit Fours

Trusting to form a few customs made eatable endowments that are beyond any doubt to inspire? Make petit fours. Including confetti cake layered with raspberry stick and buttercream and secured in a glossy white coat, these dazzling scaled down cakes will charm anybody who gets them.

Fixings

CONFETTI CAKE

- Cooking splash
- 2 1/2 c. (300 g.) all-purpose flour
- 1 1/2 tsp. preparing powder
- 3/4 tsp. legitimate salt
- 1 3/4 c. (350 g.) granulated sugar
- 1 c. (2 sticks) unsalted butter, relaxed
- 1/2 c. (4 oz.) cream cheese, relaxed
- 4 huge eggs, room temperature

- 1 tbsp. almond extricate
- 1/3 c. (80 mL.) entirety drain
- 1/2 c. rainbow sprinkles
- BUTTERCREAM
- 3/4 c. (1 1/2 sticks) unsalted butter, room temperature
- 1/4 tsp. legitimate salt
- 1 1/2 tsp. unadulterated vanilla extricate
- 1 1/2 c. (180 g.) confectioners' sugar, partitioned
- Gathering
- 3/4 c. raspberry stick
- 2/3 c. corn syrup
- 16 1/2 c. (1,980 g.) confectioners' sugar
- 5 tsp. almond extricate
- 1/2 tsp. legitimate salt
- Nourishment coloring, for icing (discretionary)

Bearings

CONFETTI CAKE

Step 1

Preheat broiler to 350°. Shower 2 (13"-by-9") metal container with cooking shower and line with material, clearing out an overhang on both long sides. In a huge bowl, whisk flour, preparing powder, and salt.

Step 2

Within the expansive bowl of a stand blender fitted with the paddle connection (or in another expansive bowl employing a handheld blender), beat granulated sugar, butter, and cream cheese on medium speed until smooth, around 1 minute. Increment speed to medium-high and proceed to defeat until white and cushy, 2 to 3 minutes more. Include eggs one at a time, beating on medium after each expansion, until joined, at that point include almond extricate and beat until combined (blend may see coagulated).

Step 3

Include drain and half of dry fixings and beat on moo speed fair until combined. Employing an elastic spatula, overlay in remaining dry fixings and sprinkles.

Step 4

Partition player between arranged container, spreading with a balanced spatula or the back of a spoon to smooth best.

Step 5

Heat cake until risen and firm to the touch, 15 to 20 minutes. Let cool to room temperature, almost 20 minutes, at that point refrigerate until cold, approximately 20 minutes longer.

Step 6

Make Ahead:

Cakes can be made 1 day ahead. Let cool, at that point wrap with plastic wrap and refrigerate.

BUTTERCREAM

In a medium bowl, employing a handheld blender on medium-high speed, beat butter and salt until smooth and velvety, around 1 miniature. Add vanilla and half of confectioners' sugar and beat until smooth, at that point include remaining confectioners' sugar and proceed to defeat until light and feathery, 2 to 3 minutes more. Set aside until prepared to utilize.

Get together

Step 1

Line a heating sheet with material. Evacuate chilled cakes from container and peel off material. Put 1 cake on arranged sheet and spread best with stick. Organize moment cake over beat side down, at that point spread top with buttercream. Refrigerate stacked cake until strong, at slightest 30 minutes or up to overnight.

Step 2

Transfer stacked cake to a cutting board. Employing a sharp chef's cut, trim 1/2" off each brief side and 1/2" off each long side. Cut cake into around 12 (1"-wide) strips. Pivot cutting board 90° (so long sides of strips are confronting you). Using a serrated cut and little delicate sawing movements, cut each strip into 7 to 8 (1") squares. Put squares on a parchment-lined heating sheet and solidify at slightest 30 minutes some time recently coating.

Step 3

In the meantime, set a wire rack interior a large preparing sheet. Fill a medium pot with 1" water and warm over medium warm until stewing, then remove from warm.

Step 4

Set a huge heatproof bowl over pot of hot water (bowl shouldn't touch water) and whisk corn syrup and 1 1/4 glasses hot water in bowl until corn syrup is broken up. Whisk in confectioners' sugar until a smooth, thick, pourable consistency shapes (blend ought to be thick, but in case it's as well thick, include more hot water, 1 tablespoon at a time, until the required consistency is come to). Whisk in almond extract and salt.

Step 5

On the off chance that craved, exchange 1/2 glass warmed coat to a little bowl and add nourishment coloring. Exchange coat to a channeling sack fitted with a little circular tip.

Step 6

Evacuate petit fours from fridge. Put one of the petit fours on a level opened spatula or angle spatula. Holding over coat bowl, spoon coat over until secured. Set coated petit four on arranged rack. Rehash with remaining petit fours. (In case coat begins to cool and solidify, turn on warm beneath pot and whisk until it comes to the required consistency. On the off chance that this doesn't work and it appears to dry out, include hot water, 1 teaspoon at a time, until desired consistency is come to.) Sprinkle coated petit fours with saved colored coat, in the event that craved.

Step 7

Let icing set until firm, at that point store in an air proof holder in the fridge.

71. Bunny Cake

Need to require your Easter dessert table to the another level? This noteworthy bunny cake looks like it came from a pastry kitchen, but is really so direct to form. It begins with a super-moist carrot cake (what else?), imaginatively cut, iced, and brightened with Easter sweet to see like a cute bunny. Permit yourself the time to truly take after the steps and have fun with the decorations—you and your occasion visitors will be so "hoppy" you did!

Fixings

CAKE

- Cooking splash
- 3/4 c. (160 g.) pressed light brown sugar or dim brown sugar
- 1/2 c. neutral oil
- 1/4 c. (50 g.) granulated sugar
- 2 huge eggs
- 1/2 tsp. unadulterated vanilla extricate
- 1 1/4 c. (150 g.) all-purpose flour

- 1 tsp. preparing powder
- 1 tsp. ground cinnamon
- 1/2 tsp. baking soda
- 1/2 tsp. ground ginger
- 1/4 tsp. legitimate salt
- 1/8 tsp. ground nutmeg
- 1 c. (110 g.) grated carrots (from almost 2 expansive)
- Icing & Brightening
- 1 1/2 c. (3 sticks) unsalted butter, room temperature
- 6 c. (690 g.) confectioners' sugar
- 1/4 c. (or more) overwhelming cream, room temperature
- 2 tsp. immaculate vanilla extricate
- 1/4 tsp. legitimate salt
- 4 c. (340 g.) sweetened destroyed coconut, isolated, additionally more in the event that needed
- 2 store-bought or custom made Rice Krispies Treats
- Pink sanding sugar, jam beans, and green nourishment coloring, for enhancing

Directions

CAKE

Step 1

Preheat broiler to 350°. Oil an 8" cake container with cooking shower; line foot with material.

Step 2

In a huge bowl, whisk brown sugar, oil, granulated sugar, eggs, and vanilla until combined and no protuberances stay. In a medium bowl, whisk flour, preparing powder, cinnamon, heating pop, ginger, salt, and nutmeg. Include dry fixings to brown sugar blend and crease with an elastic spatula until fair combined. Overlay in carrots. Rub hitter into arranged dish.

Step 3

Prepare cake until an analyzer inserted into the center comes out clean, 25 to 30 minutes. Let cool totally.

Icing & Brightening

Step 1

In a huge bowl, employing a handheld mixer or stand blender fitted with the paddle connection, on medium speed, beat butter until velvety, almost 1 minute. Add confectioners' sugar, cream, vanilla, and salt. Beat on moo speed to fair combine, almost 30 seconds, at that point increment speed to tall and beat, including more cream on the off chance that icing looks dry, until exceptionally velvety and fluffy, about 2 minutes.

Step 2

Evacuate cake from container and transfer to a cutting board. Cut cake down the center, making 2 half-moons. Flip one half-moon circular side down and ice level side with buttercream. Best with moment half-moon level side down. Stand cakes upright to make bunny body. Exchange bunny body to a platter.

Step 3

Cut out a 3" wedge around one-third of the way up from bottom of body, shaping the head. Trim head with a sharp or serrated cut to create a more adjusted shape, in the event that wanted. Put wedge on inverse conclusion of head and secure with 2 toothpicks, creating the tail and trimming, if craved.

Step 4

Ice whole bunny with a lean coat of buttercream (it doesn't got to be idealize, as the coconut will stow away any blemishes). Refrigerate to set, 15 to 30 minutes. Liberally ice cake once more with buttercream. Sprinkle whole bunny with 2 mugs coconut, utilizing more in case required, to cover and make hide.

Step 5

Carve out 2 ears from Rice Krispies Treats. Ice with buttercream and sprinkle interior of ears with sanding sugar. Sprinkle ears with 1 glass coconut for hide. Using toothpicks, press ears into head. Utilizing jam beans, make eyes and a nose.

Step 6

In a tightly secured jostle or holder, shake remaining 1 glass coconut with a drop of green nourishment coloring, including more nourishment coloring in the event that required, until coated and craved color is come to. Sprinkle around bunny and enhance with more jam beans.

72. Parmesan-Crusted Cabbage Steaks Are the Most Delicious Way to Eat Cabbage

These delicate cabbage steaks are brushed with balsamic vinegar and oil on both sides to assist with caramelization whereas moreover including sweetness to every bite. In the event that you have got any extra cabbage after cutting the steaks, chop it up and spare it for a serving of mixed greens, or utilize it for simmering the taking after day.

Fixings

- 1 little head green cabbage (approximately 2 pounds)
- 2 tablespoons extra-virgin olive oil

- 2 tablespoons balsamic vinegar
- 1/2 teaspoon ground pepper, separated
- 1/4 teaspoon salt
- 1/2 glass ground Parmesan cheese
- 2 teaspoons finely chopped new flat-leaf parsley, additionally more for decorate
- 1 teaspoon finely chopped new thyme
- 1/4 teaspoon paprika
- 1/4 teaspoon garlic powder
- 4 teaspoons balsamic coat (discretionary)

Headings

Step 1

Position broiler rack in lower third; preheat to 425°F. Line a huge rimmed preparing sheet with thwart. Evacuate and dispose of any free external takes off from cabbage; trim root conclusion and cut the cabbage into 4 (1-inch-thick) steaks.

Step 2

Whisk oil, vinegar, 1/4 teaspoon pepper and salt together in a little bowl. Brush the blend equally over both sides of the cabbage steaks;

put them on the arranged heating sheet. Cook until browned on the foot, around 25 minutes, pivoting the container from front to back midway through.

Step 3

In the meantime, combine Parmesan, parsley, thyme, paprika, garlic powder and the remaining 1/4 teaspoon pepper in a little bowl; mix well.

Step 4

Evacuate the preparing sheet from the stove. Employing a adaptable metal spatula, carefully flip the cabbage steaks. Sprinkle the Parmesan blend equitably over the tops of the steaks (almost 2 tablespoons each).

Step

Cook until the cabbage is delicate and the cheese blend is brilliant brown, 10 to 12 minutes, pivoting the heating sheet from front to back midway through.

Drizzle with balsamic coat, if using, and embellish with extra parsley, in the event that wanted.

GLUTEN-FREE Pastries

73. Gluten-Free Ice Cream Sandwiches

No offense to the Chipwich, but nothing compares to a classic ice cream sandwich the kind with delicate rectangular chocolate treats on both closes. This formula is gluten-free, keto-friendly, and fair as delicious as the notorious store-bought treats you developed up with.

Ingredients

- Cooking splash
- 3/4 c. unsweetened cocoa powder
- 2/3 c. almond flour
- 2/3 c. Swerve confectioners
- 1 tsp. heating pop

- 3/4 tsp. legitimate salt
- 1/2 c. (1 adhere) butter, softened
- 2 expansive eggs
- 3 c. keto-friendly ice cream

Headings

Step 1

Preheat broiler to 350°. Line a expansive heating sheet with material paper and oil with cooking splash. In a huge bowl, whisk together cocoa powder, almond flour, sweetener, preparing pop, and salt. Include softened butter and eggs and whisk until fair combined. Utilizing a balanced spatula, spread player into an indeed layer on arranged heating sheet.

Step 2

Heat until scarcely set and a toothpick inserted in middle comes out clean, about 7 minutes. Let cool totally.

Step 3

Line another expansive preparing sheet with material paper, at that point flip cooled cookie onto it. Cut in half widthwise.

Step 4

Let ice cream sit until relaxed marginally, at that point spread over one half utilizing a balanced spatula. To assist spread ice cream, run your counterbalanced beneath hot water and wipe off with a paper towel. Utilize material to assist flip the other half on best and press to create beyond any doubt it is sandwiched well. Solidify until totally strong, at slightest 4 hours.

Step 5

Cut into 24 squares that are 2x2-inch each and keep in cooler until prepared to serve.

74. Gluten-Free Apple Pie

I trust you're not batting your eyes at "gluten-free." So regularly is the word related with negative essences since there's fair nothing very like a gluten-filled treat bread, pasta, pie, cakes, treats, you title it… or so you think. Halt there:

Gluten-free apple pie can be fair as great as all the others. It's approximately utilizing the proper flour, parcels of butter, including fair sufficient water, and having persistence.

Fixings

Batter

- 1 1/2 c. (220 g.) gluten-free flour, such as Bob's Ruddy Process Gluten-Free 1 to 1 flour
- 1 c. (120 g.) stone-ground white cornmeal
- 1 tbsp. granulated sugar
- 1/4 tsp. legitimate salt
- 1 c. (2 sticks) cold unsalted butter, cut into cubes
- 3/4 c. ice cold water
- FILLING & Gathering
- 3 Pink Lady apples (about 400 g.), peeled, cored, and meagerly cut
- 3 Granny Smith apples (about 400 g.), peeled, cored, and daintily cut
- 3/4 c. (150 g.) granulated sugar
- 1/2 c. (55 g.) cornstarch
- 1/4 c. (45 g.) new lemon juice
- 1 tsp. ground cinnamon
- Squeeze of legitimate salt
- Cooking shower
- Gluten-free flour, for tidying

- 1 huge egg
- 1 tbsp. turbinado sugar

Bearings

Batter

Step 1

In an expansive bowl, whisk flour, cornmeal, granulated sugar, and salt. Utilizing your fingertips, blend butter into dry fixings until huge pea-size pieces' frame. Include water and blend with a fork until combined.

Step 2

Turn out mixture onto a work surface and separate in half. Gently work each half fair until mixture comes together. Press to a disk, making beyond any doubt no scraps stay.

Step 3

Wrap disks in plastic wrap. Refrigerate at slightest 30 minutes or up to 24 hours.

FILLING & Gathering

Step 1

In a large bowl, hurl apples, granulated sugar, cornstarch, lemon juice, cinnamon, and salt until coated.

Step 2

Let 1 disk of mixture rest at room temperature 10 minutes. Oil a 9" pie dish with cooking shower. Liberally tidy work surface with flour (the batter is exceptionally delicate and delicate, so it'll be difficult to work with in case it sticks).

Step 3

Roll batter to a circular 11" to 12" in breadth approximately 1/8" thick. Tenderly overlay dough into quarters. Exchange to arranged dish (in case batter breaks, squeeze it back together). Unfurl mixture and solidly press against sides and foot of skillet. Trim, clearing out almost 1" overhang. Pour filling into mixture.

Step 4

Softly clean work surface with more flour. Roll remaining disk of mixture to a circular 11" in breadth almost 1/8" to 1/4" thick. Gently crease mixture into quarters and put over filling. Unfurl mixture, at that point trim edges of best circular, taking off a 1/2" overhang. Overlay edge of foot circular up and over; press together to seal. Utilizing your list finger and thumb from one hand and your file finger from the other, make little spaces around edges. Refrigerate until chilled, about 30 minutes.

Step 5

Orchestrate a rack in lower third of stove; preheat to 400°. Cut a small X in beat of pie. In a little bowl, beat egg with a sprinkle of water until mixed. Brush beat and edges of pie with egg wash. Sprinkle with turbinado sugar.

Step 6

Prepare pie 30 minutes. Diminish stove temperature to 375° and proceed to prepare until hull is brilliant brown, around 30 minutes longer.

Step 7

Let cool about 20 minutes some time recently cutting.

75. **Gluten-Free Brownies**

Keep in mind those Small Debbie Infinite Brownies with the rainbow chocolate chips? Those were on my intellect whereas making these gluten-free squares of cocoa enchant. Allowed, presently that I'm not within the fourth review, I exchanged out the rainbow chips for some chopped hazelnuts if you are a partner of Nutella, you'll adore this blending. In case you're unfavorably susceptible or fair not a fan of nuts, feel free to skip it the brownie will taste fair as great.

Fixings

- 3/4 c. grapeseed oil
- 3/4 c. dutch handle cocoa
- 1 1/2 c. common cocoa
- 1 tsp. legitimate salt
- 1/4 tsp. heating powder
- 5 huge egg whites
- 1 2/3 c. granulated sugar
- 1 tsp. immaculate vanilla extract
- 1/4 c. chopped hazelnuts (discretionary)

Headings

Step 1

Preheat broiler to 325°. Oil a 9"-x-9" preparing container with cooking splash, line with material, at that point oil with cooking shower once more.

Step 2

In an expansive blending bowl, whisk together cocoas. In a little pot over medium warm, warm oil to 240°, about 2 minutes. Pour hot oil over cocoa and blend to combine completely until no dry spots stay, at that point let sit for 10 minutes.

Step 3

To cocoa bowl, include salt, heating powder, and egg whites. Utilizing a hand mixer, beat until blend is fully incorporated and expansive disintegrates frame. Include sugar and vanilla and continue beating until mixture becomes totally smooth, lightened, and shiny.

Step 4

Exchange player into arranged container and smooth best, at that point sprinkle with chopped hazelnuts, in case utilizing.

Step 5

Heat until a toothpick embedded into the center comes out with some sodden pieces connected, approximately 30 minutes.

Step 6

Let cool totally some time recently cutting into squares.

76. Aperol Spritz Trifle

Once you need a show-stopping dessert, there are few dishes that are as wonderful as a play. This old-school English dessert dates back as early as the 16th century as a way to utilize up stale pieces of cake. Whereas the beginnings of a play are quite humble, they've advanced to gotten to be more expand over a long time. The substituting layers of cake, cream, custard, natural product, and indeed gelatin are implied to not as it were taste debauched, but too see outwardly dazzling.

Fixings

CAKE

- Cooking splash
- 1 (15.25-oz.) box vanilla cake, also fixings called for on box
- 1/2 c. Prosecco
- Pizzazz of 1 orange
- PUDDING
- 1 (3.4-oz.) box instant vanilla pudding, additionally ingredients called for on box

- 3 tbsp. Aperol
- WHIPPED CREAM
- 1 1/2 c. overwhelming cream
- 1 tbsp. confectioners' sugar
- 1 tsp. unadulterated vanilla extricate
- APEROL Stick
- 1 c. apricot jam
- 2 tbsp. Aperol

Bearings

CUPCAKES

Step 1

Preheat stove to temperature recorded in bundle enlightening. Oil a standard 12-cup muffin tin with cooking shower.

Step 2

In a medium bowl, combine cake mix, ingredients called for on box, supplanting 1/2 container water with Prosecco, and orange zest until well combined. Separate player among arranged biscuit glasses.

Step 3

Heat cupcakes until an analyzer embedded into the center comes out clean, 20 to 23 minutes. Let cool. Expel cakes from mugs and exchange to a cutting board. Cut each in half parallel to work surface.

www.ingramcontent.com/pod-product-compliance
Lightning Source LLC
Chambersburg PA
CBHW062102220526
45471CB00010B/3570